T0208948

Front and back cover photo:

"Forget-me-not" (Myosotis Alpestris) Location: Lower Saddle of The Grand Teton, Grand Teton National Park, Wyoming, elevation 11,500ft.

Photo: Isa Oehry©

HEALING LYME BEYOND ANTIBIOTICS

A PERSONAL ACCOUNT OF WINNING THE BATTLE
AGAINST LYME DISEASE

ISABELLA S. OEHRY

BALBOA.PRESS
A DIVISION OF HAY HOUSE

Balboa Press books may be ordered through
booksellers or by contacting:

Balboa Press
A Division of Hay House
1663 Liberty Drive
Bloomington, IN 47403
www.balboapress.com
1 (877) 407-4847

Print information available on the last page.

ISBN: 978-1-9822-3922-0 (sc)
ISBN: 978-1-9822-3923-7 (e)

Balboa Press rev. date: 02/10/2020

CONTENTS

PART I   MY STORY

PART II   TICKS AND LYME SPIROCHETES

PART III TREATMENTS

FOREWORD

by Timothy Lee Scott

"Stories are a pharmacopoeia, a
storehouse of culture and wisdom.
Not only are they food for the soul. They
are medicine for the soul as well."

Jon Kabat-Zinn, Forward to *Soul Food: Stories
to Nourish the Spirit and the Heart*
by Jack Kornfield & Christina Feldman

Isa has a story to tell. A personal account of illness and
healing, along with tales of plants and animals, insects
and bacteria, and the whole of the natural world around
us. It's a story of the interconnectedness of all things, the
intermingling of different forms of life.

This book shares how bacteria can hitch a ride in the
gut of an insect, which then hops onto an animal and
latches on, allowing the bacteria to stealthily move through
species, infecting, feeding and reproducing, causing havoc
and despair in those humans unlucky enough to become a
host to this unwelcomed guest. Fortunately, there are plants
that are likely growing right outside your door that can help.

This is a tale of hope and recovery.

When Isa asked me to come and give a talk at her place, it had been a few years since I had publicly spoke, and had forgotten how important it was that I go out and share my story. Personal tales of our own suffering can allow others to realize they are not alone, and this in itself can be healing, and relax those tensions from feeling isolated. It obviously moved Isa enough to include it in her book you now hold, and I feel it is an important tale to tell, with a unique perspective. Just as Isa has her own unique experience to share, with her battle with Lyme disease.

This is a cautionary tale of the failure of conventional Western medicine.

Since 2004, when I was first introduced to Lyme disease and treating it with natural remedies, I have met and heard from thousands of individuals who have a similar story to tell as Isa. Unfortunately, it has often been a barrage of misdiagnoses, mistreatments, and debilitating symptoms, which can utterly destroy a person's life. They have been to countless doctors, been told they have numerous diseases, treated with questionable methods, and if lucky enough to have a positive Lyme test, then subjected to a multitude of antibiotics which don't often hit their intended target.

Fortunately, there are pioneers in the Lyme terrain that have been able to think outside the box and get up close and personal with the Lyme bacterium. Those who have gotten to know *Borrelia burgdorferi* cannot help but be in awe of this organism, who is both intelligent and conscious, and has learned ways to infect and highjack a person's body, out-maneuvering the innate immune system. It has adapted to the onslaught of antibiotics, learned to change form, and lay dormant for years on end if need be. It has the ability to penetrate deep into the body, cloak itself, becoming a "master of elusiveness" and then mimic other diseases and disorders, making it difficult to diagnose, becoming a "great impostor" and disguising its true identity. By looking this way and getting to know this organism, it takes away the mystery that can cripple the mind, and allows us to see it for what it is.

With Isa's personal experience and her investigation into Lyme disease, she has seen this world up close and has the experience to guide others through the terrain, just as she might lead others climbing the Grand Teton mountains.

After treating Lyme disease for many years, and then suffering with it myself, I have found the most important medicine for people who are ill, is hope. This book provides that remedy.

--Timothy Lee Scott

Preface

"Health is the crown on the well person's head
that only the ill person can see."

—Robin Sharma

During the summer of 2016 Western medicine failed me. Unable to cure me with antibiotics, the standard treatment for Lyme disease, neurologists predicted chronic, long-term and potentially debilitating symptoms down the road. Yet, they were not able to offer any different treatment for the future. When the downward spiral of Lyme disease became unbearable, more aggressive rounds of antibiotics that required intravenous delivery would be prescribed. Sick, miserable, and unwilling to take more antibiotics, I began searching for alternative methods to cure myself.

I had absolutely no idea, when I embarked on this fascinating road of discovery, where the research would take me. I learned of powerful natural remedies that are capable of reducing Lyme disease symptoms, even offering a full recovery, as I have experienced. I discovered mind-boggling facts about the super intelligent bacteria that cause the disease. And, believe it or not, I even began to marvel at the unusual lives and capabilities of ticks, the main culprits these days when it comes to infecting humans with *Borrelia burgdorferi*.

During my research, the number of people I came in contact with who either suffer from Lyme disease, or know someone who does, was staggering. People had often been ill for years and had sometimes gone through several unsuccessful rounds of antibiotics. They felt discouraged and, tragically, believed that there was no hope for ever recovering their health.

I feared that, without the knowledge of alternative treatments and unaware that a road to recovery exists, these people would continue to suffer and only get worse. I had to share my experience.

Ultimately, it was the failure of antibiotic treatments that inspired me to begin my research. And it was my gradual and eventual recovery that was the catalyst to begin writing this book. My hope is that *Healing Lyme Beyond Antibiotics* may be of help to you as well, or to those you know who suffer from this disease.

ACKNOWLEDGEMENTS

I embarked on this journey desperately searching for alternative methods to heal myself from Lyme disease after a failed treatment with antibiotics. At the time, I knew very little about the disease. It was only due to the diligent study and meticulous records of those who dedicate their lives to healing that I was able to find pertinent information and, ultimately, a cure for myself. I am deeply grateful to these wonderful people who have kept the wisdom of plant medicine alive.

My deepest gratitude, hands down, goes to Stephen Harrod Buhner. Although I have never met Buhner personally, his extensive work on Lyme disease was invaluable to my recovery. Buhner has studied Lyme disease for over thirty-five years. He has written several books on healing Lyme and many other books on related topics. I consider Buhner an absolute authority on healing Lyme and a genius when it comes to understanding the healing power of plants. I recommend his book *Healing Lyme* to anyone interested in learning about Lyme *Borreliosis*, its coinfections, the body's intricate system of defense, the bacteria involved, and why certain treatments work and others don't.

I am tremendously grateful to Timothy Lee Scott, a most compassionate and knowledgeable practitioner who specializes in treating Lyme disease. Tim's background is in Chinese medicine, acupuncture, and herbalism. He is also a writer and researcher and shares his knowledge about plants and their healing power in his book *Invasive Plant Medicine*. It was no surprise that my research about herbal remedies for Lyme disease would eventually lead to Tim. I had the pleasure of meeting Tim personally and am touched to this day by his compassion and willingness to help those afflicted with Lyme disease.

I am deeply grateful to Grace Johnstone, DC, for sharing so generously her personal story. Much of the information in the chapter "Hyperbaric Chamber: Oxygen Therapy" was contributed by Grace. It is because of outstanding people like her that professionals in the field of healthcare, as well as the public, become aware of the tremendous benefits of this treatment modality. As her story shows, it is a powerful tool when it comes to treating and healing Lyme disease.

My deepest and heartfelt gratitude goes out to my niece Valentina Oehry. It was Valentina, an avid believer in all things natural, who suggested that I try an alternative route to cure myself of Lyme disease. Were it not for her advice, who knows where I would be today and in what condition. Her suggestion also prompted my journey into research about all Lyme-related topics, which became the foundation of this book.

I am very grateful to David Allen, professor of biology at Middlebury College, for so willingly sharing his tremendous knowledge about ticks and tick-borne diseases. David, an ecologist, studies the ecological, environmental, climatic, and landscape factors that contribute to tick populations. He researches the maintenance of tick-borne diseases in tick populations and tests these populations for the bacteria that cause Lyme disease and anaplasmosis. He is one of those rare people who are able to present this somewhat sobering information with humor and enthusiasm.

I am tremendously grateful to Dorothy Gannon, my talented editor. In her gentle and tactful ways, she continues to help me to refine my words and the skill of writing along with everything else that goes with the writing of a book without ever taking away my own voice. I value her patience and attention to detail, but above all, I most value our friendship.

I am deeply indebted to Joni B. Cole, a tremendously talented writing instructor and a dear friend. During our writing workshops, I have witnessed the many times when Joni gently nudged a writer to the next level. Joni's feedback is consistently professional, positive, and supportive. And with just a few words she can open a new world to us writers and help transform a piece of ordinary writing into something truly special.

My gratitude goes out to the many dedicated researchers, biologists, ecologists, practitioners, and authors who have so willingly shared and continue to share their wisdom.

I am also deeply grateful to the plants that have so generously assisted me in my recovery. Their "wisdom," which was built upon millions of years of experience in coexisting with bacteria, has aided my young and, in comparison, inexperienced immune system to learn and to expand.

And lastly, I am grateful to all the people I have come in contact with during my research. Everyone seems to know someone who is afflicted with Lyme disease and who struggles to get well. You reaffirmed to me again and again how desperately we need to know more about alternative treatments. And you gave me the incentive to continue my search and my writing to ultimately present you with this book.

DISCLAIMER

If you suffer from Lyme disease or suspect that you have been infected, it is best to consult a knowledgeable practitioner who is familiar with treatment modalities for alleviating Lyme symptoms and eliminating the bacteria in your body.

Healing Lyme beyond Antibiotics is a personal account. What is shared is meant to serve for informational purposes only. In no way is any information contained in this book intended as medical advice.

When microorganisms enter a body, they find a unique ecosystem that is different from any other body, and a unique immune system specific to that particular body. Once inside the body, the bacteria quickly adjust to their new host and adapt accordingly in order to secure a high rate of survival. Therefore, Lyme disease has a way of showing symptoms that vary from person to person. Pharmaceuticals or herbs that work for one person may not work for another person. What was effective for me cannot guarantee the same results for you.

With Lyme disease spreading rapidly, existing treatment methods are being adjusted and new ones developed as we speak. Our understanding about how to treat Lyme disease is constantly broadening. What is presented in this book by no means represents a complete list of available treatments but rather a recollection of what has assisted me in gaining full recovery.

DEDICATION

Healing Lyme Beyond Antibiotics
is dedicated to all who suffer from the disease.

My deepest wish is that you may find within this book
a glimmer of hope and a thread of light
guiding you to your own successful recovery.

"The world breaks every 'one'
and afterward many are strong at the broken places."

--Ernest Hemingway

PART I

MY STORY

"The wound is the place where the Light enters you."

--Rumi

Besides the inability of traditional antibiotic treatments to cure my Lyme disease, Western medicine predicted chronic and potentially debilitating effects down the road. Yet it offered no prospect for future treatments other than additional and more aggressive rounds of antibiotics that included intravenous delivery. Western medicine had failed me.

The failure of antibiotic treatments and my struggle and ultimate success in recuperating from this debilitating disease were the catalysts for my writing this book. Part I of this book will give you a glimpse into my personal experience with Lyme disease.

If you are looking specifically for information on how to treat Lyme disease with the use of nonconventional methods, skip this section and go straight to Part III, Treatments. You can always return later to find out what happened to me.

INFECTED UNBEKNOWNST

"You must return to a lower elevation," I urged Nick. We had climbed to approximately eleven thousand feet. Despite his most wholehearted efforts, the altitude strictly forbade him to climb yet another foot. He suffered terribly, getting sick all over the precious Alpine flora––missile projector style. It was not a pretty sight.

We were on the grueling path leading up to the Grand Teton when the summit became unattainable to Nick––at least for now. This peak is called "the Grand" for good reason. Located in the Grand Teton National Park in Wyoming, it towers magnificently over its neighbors at a height of 13,776 feet. It is surrounded by several other mighty peaks. Climbing the Grand, however, is particularly challenging, as there are no shortcuts. To summit many fourteen-thousand footers outside of the Teton range, one can sometimes drive a vehicle up to twelve thousand feet and then proceed from there on foot. But in the Tetons the trail begins at a plateau situated at an altitude of six thousand feet. The drastic change in altitude from six thousand to almost fourteen thousand feet cannot be tolerated by many, causing them to suffer from altitude sickness. This makes the ascent of the Grand particularly challenging for folks with a tendency to altitude sickness.

With a face the color of ash, deeply disappointed with his body so unwilling to cooperate, Nick encouraged me to go on. He was aware that it was my third attempt at this beautiful and magnificent peak and that I was feeling strong and eager to attempt the summit. After wishing me well, Nick turned around and began his descent. There is no other remedy for altitude sickness than to retreat as quickly as possible to a lower elevation. Knowing how hard this was for him, I appreciated his support and encouragement even more.

I continued alone. My plan was, now without a climbing partner, to join another team higher up. Despite the unexpected change of events, I was still driven to fulfill my lifelong dream of standing on top of the Grand.

As the air became thinner, stingy with oxygen, my body labored hard. Every step seemed a challenge to gain another foot of altitude. Yet I pushed on. Gradually, the trail became more difficult, interspersed with large tricky rock outcroppings, each of which had to be surmounted. A slip could result in serious injury. Caution was in order.

Finally, I reached the spot where the relatively easy mountaineering ends. It is here on the Upper Saddle, at an elevation of thirteen thousand feet, that climbers rope up for safety. This was the point where I had planned to join a team. To my dismay, nobody was in sight.

I stood alone, staring into the gaping abyss of the Valhalla Canyon, which loomed thousands of feet below. Its void seemed to suck me in like a powerful magnet. I had to force my eyes away to scan the rock above, searching for the climbing route.

Not used to climbing without a partner or the safety of a rope, I took my time to hatch a plan. With a sober and humble attitude, I went about studying the features of the famous Owen-Spalding route and its notorious start––the belly crawl traverse. The technical difficulties of the route were not the issue––I knew I could handle them. It was the sheer exposure that could rattle the nerves. There would be no room for mistakes, no way to recover from a hold should it break. One misstep or slip of the hand, and the precious gift of life would be wasted.

I focused on the cliff ahead and imagined each move I would make. In my mind I went over the sections higher up on the climb, the sections I could not see from my vantage point, but which I vaguely remembered from a description in the climbing guide. I broke each challenge down into small problems. I felt confident that I could master them if

I kept my poise. Finally, I made a decision. I was going to solo the route.

I started, hesitantly at first, placing just one foot out on the rock while squeezing a hand into a crack. The first step onto a sheer cliff is always the hardest. But the solid rock and the positive footing gave me confidence. I let go with my other hand and stepped out with the other foot, leaving the safety of horizontal ground behind. Now I was glued to the face of the mountain like a fly stuck to a wall. No longer was I connected to the relative safety of the Upper Saddle. There was a feeling of nothingness below me. I knew I had the option to reverse the move and return to horizontal ground. Instead, I began moving upward, slowly at first, then more assertively, while keeping a laser-sharp focus. I strictly resisted the urge of looking down between my legs into the dark void of the Valhalla Canyon.

Section by section I tackled the route, my mind on nothing else but each move I was about to make. I loved the freedom of climbing without a rope. My body moved smoother, quicker, and was lighter for the lack of protective gear which usually hangs off my climbing belt. Halfway up the climb, I worked my way through the Owen Chimney. The Chimney was treacherous as it was iced over. Not anticipating these conditions, I carried no ice axes or crampons. Luckily, I found dry rock and was able to climb around the ice.

The higher I climbed, the more energy I had. No signs of fatigue or altitude plagued me. I felt free as a bird. When I reached the upper, often slippery plates just below the peak, I rushed over them with anticipation. I had waited so long for this moment. Within seconds I was on the summit ridge, heading for the peak. With each step the ground above me became narrower until there was only one large block of rock left to climb on to. It was the very tallest point of the Grand and marked with a geological survey marker. There was no place higher to climb.

Standing on top of the peak, I stretched my arms wide and turned around and around in a circle. There was nothing taller as far as my eyes could see. I felt as if standing on the top of the world. I had climbed the Grand all by myself––or so I thought at the time. I would find out differently soon enough.

How It All Began

Scaling this mountain had been a childhood dream. While growing up surrounded by the beautiful Alps in my home country of Liechtenstein, I had seen a picture of the Grand Teton Range in an old-fashioned wall calendar. Already a lover of mountains, I instantly fell in love with the beauty of this majestic range. How amazed I would have been, then only a wide-eyed twelve-year-old, had I known that I would live in the United States later in life and summit the Grand one day.

The turbulent teenage years did not manage to sidetrack me from my love for the mountains. I spent as many Sunday mornings sleeping off the previous night's dance party as I did waking my father before dawn and begging him to give me a ride to the foot of a mountain. Equipped with a thermos of tea, a piece of bread, and a *Landjäger*––a traditional sausage––I set out to climb one of our local peaks to spend time in solitude at its top. I loved every minute of it. At the end of the day, I'd make my way back down and hitchhike home.

Not until I was twenty-one years old did I meet the two men who would become my rock-climbing teachers, mentors, and lifelong friends, one fifteen years and the other twenty-two years my senior. I remember well my very first technical climb in the Alps with them. I wore hard-soled leather hiking boots and knickerbockers, and sported long fingernails, which were painted a deep and sexy red. During that first climb, something in me caught fire. It did not take long to trade the hiking boots for climbing shoes, the knickerbockers for colorful tights, and to file back the nails, red paint no longer necessary. Rock climbing had become my passion.

My two new friends and I spent every free moment in the mountains, they leaving their wives at home and referring to me sometimes as "Fritz" to assure marital peace. If there was not enough time to climb a mountain, we met at various small rock outcroppings where we climbed after work until dark. And when it rained, we often climbed underneath an overhang until we were too cold or too wet to continue. Then we routinely headed for a coffeehouse in a nearby village and indulged in delicious pastries.

My new passion did bring with it—besides the possibility of really pissing off someone's wife—another dark threat, unbeknownst to us all. It was a danger so tiny, with a timing and striking point so entirely unpredictable, none of us could see it coming.

Rock climbing requires crawling through the bushes to get to cliffs. We were used to coming home covered in dirt and with the occasional hitchhiker—a tick. We had even named one of our favorite cliffs the "tick cliff" because we often returned home with several of these unsightly beasts buried into our skin, already bloated from sucking blood. A shower with a tick check in every crevice of the body was mandatory. We had tricks to get them off too. One of them was applying butter to the tick and gently rotating the critter counterclockwise. Eventually it would let go, its head still attached. Bizarre as it sounds, somehow it worked. (See also Part II, Tick Removal, for the recommended ways to remove ticks.)

During those years in the Alps I removed countless ticks from my body, some buried deeper into my skin than others. Not until my friend's young wife became mysteriously ill for months on end and eventually landed in the hospital, diagnosed with Lyme meningitis, did we realize and understand the danger.

Luckily, my friend's wife recuperated. But other people around us, often nonclimbers, suddenly fell ill with Lyme disease. Alarmed, we avoided "tick cliff" and became even more diligent about checking our bodies after climbing. Despite our efforts checking for ticks during and after climbing, we brought home an occasional specimen.

I removed dozens of them from my body over the years without ever getting ill.

Eventually, the turns and twists of my life landed me in the United States. I settled in Vermont and continued my passion for rock climbing with whomever was able and willing. Vermont is not quite like Switzerland or Liechtenstein, not even if drunk, delirious, or just wishful. Wherever you look, you see rolling hills––the green mountains of Vermont––covered in deciduous forests. These forests are breathtakingly beautiful. Leaf peepers from all over the world arrive each year to peek at the multicolored tree canopies during the fall. And, of course, the leaf litter is home to billions of insects, including ticks.

In the absence of large cliffs, I turned to smaller rock outcroppings to enjoy an occasional climbing experience. But I also loved hiking, biking, trail running, and more often than not simply strolling through these wonderful forests and lingering under their canopies. I treasured the smell of the earth, sometimes lying on the forest floor in the midst of ferns five feet tall, or climbing a tree to enjoy a particular view. Occasionally, but very rarely, I found a tick on myself. I simply removed it and never worried about it.

It was not until 2010, when I began climbing at a small cliff in New Hampshire, that ticks became a major issue again. That particular cliff, as much as my climbing friends and I loved it, was infested with ticks. We were more annoyed at their presence than fearful. Mandatory tick checks were back. Often, we removed several of them after a visit to the cliff. Before stepping into the car, we changed our clothing in the parking lot, inspected each piece, shook it vigorously, and then threw it into a garbage bag. At home, we transported the contents of the bag straight to the dryer in the hope that any sneaky tick hiding in the seams would be successfully fried.

We tested their behavior too. My climbing partner Nick, thoroughly grossed out by ticks, taped his climbing pants to his shoes with duct tape in order to inhibit any ticks from crawling up his legs. I can assure you, he made for a very funny sight. I went the opposite direction and hiked to the cliff in shorts and sandals so I could see and feel the attackers. Generally, I had fewer ticks, often none, if I were bare legged, while he seemed to pick them up with his clothing. We noticed that they came in waves, attacking hard in the spring, then hiding somewhere over the hot and muggy summer months, only to make another strong appearance during the fall. Their presence was also irregular from one year to the next. One spring could be almost unbearable, whereas the following year many fewer ticks were present. Just when we thought they had finally died out or moved somewhere else, the blood suckers would be back in full force.

I never got sick from tick bites. My health and stamina were great. If these ticks were infected by a disease, the disease did not affect me.

Everything Changed

May of 2016 found me at a hospital for a checkup. I had injured my finger. The injury had gotten infected and required surgery. My surgeon, a terrific and talented Southern lady, declared the procedure a success. My finger had healed nicely and mobility promised to return to normal after a little more time and a few silly but effective exercises.

During this hospital visit, I was running a fever and felt extremely weak and achy. This concerned the surgeon. I reasoned with her that I probably had picked up a late springtime flu. Suspicious, she insisted that I not leave the hospital until I was seen by a general practitioner. Reluctantly, I complied.

In the absence of my primary caregiver, another practitioner gave me a thorough up and down. I had noticed a couple of days prior to my visit that the lymph nodes in my left groin area were swollen and extremely painful. I had also discovered a small brown mark in the same area, no larger than the size of a poppy seed. I suggested that the spot could well be the mark of a spider bite. We have some nasty creepy crawlers in Vermont, such as the black widow or the brown recluse, which can't kill you but can cause symptoms that make you want to run and seek medical attention.

Even though I exhibited no classic bullseye rash, I did mention that a tick bite should not be ruled out because of my love of roaming in the woods. The practitioner took note of my concern and stated that she would order a Lyme disease test, together with an entire array of blood tests to get to the bottom of things. She also scheduled me for an ultrasound of my uterus and urged me to consider a CAT scan as she suspected a serious illness gnawing at my life.

Perplexed, I returned home to rest. The hospital would call with results of the blood test within a few days. After a week I was back to normal and happy to have a fully functioning finger that finally allowed me to climb again.

I was annoyed at having to undergo the ultrasound and simply refused the CAT scan. Plus, I had planned an extended trip out West with my climbing partner Nick. The itinerary of our trip included many exciting climbing adventures. Our starting date was set for mid-June, and I was in no frame of mind to change my plans. I was feeling healthy.

In mid-June the hospital called with the lab results. It seemed that, after all, my life was not in imminent danger. No results for the Lyme disease test were available at that point. Typically, Lyme disease test results can take up to two or three weeks. I was unconcerned as I was feeling splendid and very excited about our upcoming trip. I decided to call the hospital in a week or two while on the road.

After only one week on the road, I fell ill again. I had a fever, night sweats, joint pain, and suffered extreme exhaustion. I convinced myself that the flu had lingered and was just making a reappearance. At the time, we were camped out at the bottom of Devil's Tower National Monument in Wyoming.

Not wanting to miss out on the incredible adventure of climbing Devil's Tower, I insisted on sticking to our four o'clock alpine start despite feeling miserable. That day I was unable to take the lead while climbing. In fact, I was barely able to follow Nick up the cliff. Watching me struggle, he suggested that I may have Lyme disease after all. Later that day I called the hospital again to inquire about the test results. I was informed that the results were not in yet. Within another week I felt fine.

The further west we travelled, the better I felt while enjoying our fabulous rock-climbing adventures. At Nick's insistence, however, I called the hospital again after another week on the road. We knew from climbing friends who had suffered from Lyme disease that the earlier the diagnosis the better the chances for a successful treatment. When I called the hospital, the nurse at the other end of the phone admitted that there was no trace in my records of any Lyme disease test ever being ordered. I was stunned. There was no other option but to accept the fact that there was no test and therefore no test results. It had been well over seven weeks since my initial symptoms in May, too late for a so-called early detection.

Since I was feeling good and getting stronger every day, I decided that whatever had ailed me was on its way south, so to speak. Plus, I had a routine annual checkup scheduled for August back in Vermont after our trip. I could address the issue of the missing test at that time with my primary caregiver.

For now, I decided to put my worries to rest and to enjoy the trip. We travelled from South Dakota to Wyoming, Montana, and Colorado, hiking or climbing every day to build up stamina and adjust to the altitude. Our eyes were set on the Grand Teton.

It was July when I stood at the very top of that majestic peak. While turning around and around in a circle, arms stretched wide, I thought I had the view all to myself. In a way I did, of course. But in another way, I did not know that I had thousands of companions. It would be another month before I would find out that an entire army of malicious bacteria, spirochetes named *Borrelia burgdorferi*, had conveniently hitchhiked to the peak with me.

BEGINNING OF DECLINE

When I saw my primary caregiver after our trip, I gave her a quick update on the curious events of the flu episodes and the missing Lyme disease test. She suggested that I simply take the test now to confirm that I was indeed clear of Lyme bacteria. It had been three months since the first flu-like episode. Unconcerned, I consented, gave blood, and returned home feeling healthier and stronger than ever.

Three weeks later the phone rang. It was my primary with the results of the blood test. With a hesitant voice she stated: "You are *SO* positive."

I remember pondering her choice of words. At the time I was under the impression that you could only be either positive or negative for Lyme. So, what on earth does *SO* positive mean?

As I was to find out much later, the Western blot test––the common test given for suspected Lyme disease––measures the number of antibody bands (immunoglobulin G and M) that the immune system has produced in response to the presence of Lyme bacteria in the blood. One to two bands are considered normal, as we all have some spirochetes in our body. Two to five antibody bands indicate the presence of Lyme disease bacteria and a strong immune response to fight the invaders. Two to five antibody bands are considered a positive test result for Lyme disease.

My blood test showed *ten* IgG bands and *two* IgM bands!

Not knowing anything about Lyme disease at that point and suddenly feeling extremely invaded and fearful, I agreed on the spot to the standard Lyme disease protocol that my primary caregiver suggested––a massive course of antibiotics. A full thirty days of Doxycycline.

Doxycycline over such a long period of time robbed my gut of any bacteria––good and bad. If I had not been feeling lousy before the treatment, I sure did afterwards. After a month of the stuff I was wiped out, tired, had lost weight and was achy all the time. The small hospital, unable to assist me further now that I was actually ill, referred me to specialists in the neurology department of a well-known, large hospital. During my appointment with the neurologist I was assured that it was wise to establish a relationship in the early stages of the disease, in the event that things went from bad to worse. Options such as future multiple rounds of antibiotics, including by intravenous delivery, if necessary, were discussed. I was horrified.

What followed was a long stretch of misery––not enough to be bedridden, but enough to change my life considerably. After my natural defenses were destroyed, the spirochetes found their way through the fluids of the central nervous system into my brain, where they wreaked havoc. My thinking became lethargic. I suffered from a lack of concentration. Cotton-brain is the closest I can come to describing it. My body temperature was off. Usually plenty warm and a lover of cold-water dips, I was suddenly always chilled. I was dizzy all the time. If I turned a corner, went through a doorway, or walked around a table, as if drunk I would have to grab the doorframe or the furniture to keep from keeling over. I had absolutely no balance. My eyes suffered. Within a very short time it became difficult to read, and my eyeglasses no longer worked.

Then my fingertips and toes started to sting as if a thousand needles were pricking me at the same time. I experienced burning shooting pains and numbness in my limbs. My nervous system was so hypersensitized, it would freak me out if anything touched my skin. A hair that landed on my skin would make me jump. Any touching of my body was definitely out. I was down to one and a half hours of sleep per night. I ended up bringing my pet to a friend, as the smallest noise kept me up. Any movement, too much light, too many people nearby, just about anything was too much for my racked up nervous system. I was a wreck.

Then the spirochetes found their way into my joints–– one of their favorite places to reside. My joints began to feel unnaturally loose. With my cartilage softened by their feces (yuck!) it is no surprise that I became overflexible. Soon I tore a ligament, and then my back went out. Usually a person who prefers not to use pharmaceuticals if at all possible, I pumped myself full of any medication I could find to ease the debilitating pain.

That wasn't all, however. With my immune system severely compromised, I no longer had any resistance. I could tell how hard it was for my body to fight infections. Normally, scratches and cuts would heal quickly, often overnight. Now, if I got even the smallest scratch from a blackberry bush, it would swell, hurt, ooze, and stay inflamed for weeks. Then, finally, it would calm down and begin to heal, which would take another week or two. And that just for a little scratch. I knew that if I were to get a more severe cut or injury, I would be in serious trouble.

It takes a lifetime to build up our immune system. The early years are especially crucial. With my defenses wiped out, it was exhausting for my body to keep up with the onslaught of viruses and bacteria common in our everyday surroundings. Without a healthy immune system capable of fighting off these invaders, viruses and bacteria had free range. I caught a flu that wiped me out for eight weeks.

For someone who had hardly ever been sick in her life, who was used to being strong, athletic and healthy, this was a drastic change. As my condition worsened and my ability to function decreased, a deep sadness enveloped my entire being. Nowadays, we have a term for this sadness. We call it depression. I would later find out that, not surprisingly, depression is a common side effect of Lyme disease.

The general response from the world around me was an acknowledgement that, yes, we all are getting older. And with getting older, we must accept that our bodies change. I instinctively knew, despite the fact that I was indeed getting older every day, something else was terribly wrong.

Turnaround

The turnaround began when I visited my family in Europe. My niece (all angels, saints, gods of every religion, and other heavenly beings if you do indeed exist, please bless her) suggested I try a homeopathic remedy made from a plant called *teasel*. I quickly did research and found much evidence that this plant indeed seems to have the capability to reduce symptoms of Lyme disease. Through the research I also began to learn a lot about spirochetes, the bacteria causing the disease.

First and foremost, I discovered that a healthy immune system can and will fight off spirochetes successfully without any pharmaceutical help! This explains why I had never gotten sick despite the dozens of tick bites I had experienced in Europe and later in the US. It is highly unlikely that all of these ticks had been bacteria-free. But I was healthy then and my immune system most likely able to fight off the intruders on its own.

I further learned more about the results of the Western blot test. We already know that three to five antibody bands are considered positive for Lyme disease. If many more bands are present, like the ten in my case, the results indicate that the immune system is actually working full tilt with a good chance of fighting off the invaders successfully! Spirochetes have been around for millions of years and probably have invaded humans since the beginning of mankind. The fact that I felt strong and healthy, despite being infected by the bacteria and showing a high count of antibody bands, suggests that my immune system already knew how to fight them and had been well on the way to sending them packing. Once, however, the healthy population of gut bacteria had been wiped out by the heavy and extended dose of antibiotics, the immune system was severely weakened. Spirochetes had free range to feed and to multiply.

In essence, what this means is that any progress my immune system had made prior to taking the antibiotics was wiped out through the thirty-day cycle of the drug. You can imagine how this information disturbed me and drove me further into research.

I discovered much about the microorganisms that had made me so ill. The more I learned, the more I began to respect them. They are incredibly intelligent organisms. I came to admire their capabilities, rather than to hate them for what they did to me, and I document much of what I discovered in the chapter that follows. Don't miss out on reading this chapter. I'll guarantee you, you will be amazed.

Spirochetes nibble away pretty much on anything that has low blood supply and low levels of oxygen. They favor collagen, protein from the binding tissue, tendons, fascia, ligaments, cartilage, nerve sheaths, cerebrospinal fluid, eye fluid, and so on. A healthy body easily replaces the loss of these substances without showing any symptoms. This means that a healthy body remains symptom-free despite the presence of spirochetes. This is the reason why I continued to feel strong and healthy even though spirochetes had taken residence in my body. And it explains why I was able to continue to climb mountains that required one to be in excellent shape, to have stamina, balance, and endurance.

But suddenly, there was hope. There was *teasel*. The literature promised that teasel would render the environment within the cells, where the spirochetes had taken residence, uncomfortable for the bacteria. Not happy with this change, the bacteria experience an urge to move elsewhere. In an effort to escape the discomfort, they return to the bloodstream. Here a restored immune system can fight them off successfully. Discouraged by the sudden immune response, the bacteria attempt to flee the bloodstream while exiting through the skin. When exiting through the skin, so the literature reads, itchiness would be experienced. I was hopeful, but at the same time also very doubtful. It all sounded a bit hokey-pokey and wild. But I did not see any harm in trying. I was miserable. What could I lose?

It was close to six months since the original tick bite, but I could still see the faintest mark, no larger than the prick of a pin, where the bite was. To my utter surprise, on the third day of taking the homeopathic teasel remedy, the bite mark began to swell and itch. It itched for days, followed by many more spots all over my body, which I reckoned were probably former bites of ticks or other insects.

Insects of all kinds carry bacteria. Because the transmission of spirochetes from host to host takes rather long, it is assumed that black flies, mosquitoes, horseflies, and fleas, whose bites are quick and short, are not transmitters of the bacterium. I had noticed, however, a strange phenomenon over the years. Each spring, when I was bitten by the first black flies of the season, I would experience mild cold symptoms—a light headache and a little bit of a sore throat. The symptoms always disappeared within a few days. Jokingly, I told my friends that I was allergic to black flies, nuisances we did not have in Europe. Meanwhile, I had discovered that black flies also carry *Borrelia burgdorferi* spirochetes—who would have thought?

And then there are horseflies. Their bites sting, swell, and itch. I seem to be particularly prone to attracting these buzzers. They sneak up on me while I'm jogging and with certain predictability bite my right shoulder. Why the right shoulder? I have no idea. But there must be a common understanding among horseflies about this. What is interesting, however, is that the itching of these bites never stops completely and returns at mysterious intervals. This has been going on for years. I have scars from scratching. My suspicion is that spirochetes that infiltrate my body via horsefly bites survive and remain in the area of the skin where the bite took place, hence the continuous itching in that particular area.

Usually, I was quite annoyed by the itching. After taking the teasel, however, I was thrilled with the discomfort. Something was happening. Teasel was kicking out the bacteria through the skin just as the description promised. It is recommended that one take the homeopathic teasel remedy for thirty days, to make sure that a reproductive cycle of the bacterium (which is said to happen every twenty-eight days) is covered. I was not going to give the spirochetes a chance. I took the remedy for six months straight.

After six months I was feeling considerably better. But I was not my old self––not yet. Inspired by the progress, however, I continued my research with renewed vigor. I learned that teasel indeed works very well for alleviating Lyme disease symptoms in Europe and in the Midwest of the United States. Interestingly, it is also in those areas that teasel grows plentifully. In the Northeast of the United States, where I had contracted Lyme disease, teasel does not grow. Statistics reveal that, in these areas, teasel does not seem to be as effective at eliminating Lyme disease symptoms. I needed something else.

RECOVERY

I was hot on the trail of natural remedies for curing Lyme disease. I attended talks on the subject in Europe as well as the United States, even organized informational lectures at my house. I read every book I could find about healing Lyme disease and spoke with anybody who was willing to lend an ear or share information. I was particularly interested in what natural practitioners and healers had to say.

Then I learned of an invasive species of plant that grows plentifully in the Northeast and is credited with the skill to do the magic. There indeed seems to be a correlation between bacteria and viruses, and certain plants readily available in areas where these organisms roam or grow. What is considered one of the Northeast's biggest pests is in fact a miracle plant. Its roots have the ability to suck up pollutants in the areas where it grows. Or, to put it differently, it often grows where the earth needs healing. And, kindly, it lends its healing qualities to humans as well. You can see it growing in thick bushes and clusters along riverbeds, helping to purify the water, and it is almost always found where a dump used to be, helping to clean the earth. This so-called "pest" would turn out to be my savior: Japanese knotweed.

Things come our way for reasons. As soon as I had discovered the Japanese knotweed, I came across Stephen Harrod Buhner's book *Healing Lyme*. In his book I found the missing piece of the puzzle––an herbal healing protocol. Buhner is rightfully referred to as "one of the plant geniuses of our time." In his book, Buhner puts together a core protocol consisting of a collection of medicinal plants with which to rid oneself of Lyme spirochetes. His main weapon: Japanese knotweed. I was thrilled.

Buhner's protocol is based on years of experience successfully treating thousands of people suffering from

Lyme disease. Besides the core protocol listed below, he also offers different combinations of herbal remedies for various kinds of symptoms caused by Lyme disease.

Here are the three main remedies he recommends as the core protocol:

Japanese Knotweed   (*Polygonum cuspidatum*)
Red Sage   (*Salvia miltiorrhiza*)
Chinese Scullcap   (*Scutellaria baicalensis*)

It had been roughly one year since the onset of my illness when I began taking these supplements. I took them as tinctures and eventually mixed them together into one convenient formula the way Buhner recommends. (All protocols and exact measurements I used can be found in the Appendix.)

After about three months of taking the core protocol, I added Green Chiretta (*Andrographis*) to the mix, a supplement that actually goes about killing off the *Borrelia burgdorferi* bacteria. I purposefully waited a few months before adding this remedy to allow my immune system time to get a little stronger, as caution with Green Chiretta is in order. This Chinese herb is not for everyone. It can cause an unpleasant Herxheimer reaction, which is a response to the dead bacterial fragments floating in the system before exiting. Please read more information on Herxheimer reactions in Part III, "Treatments," and be sure to read it carefully if you are considering this protocol. A Herxheimer reaction can be not only unpleasant but potentially dangerous. It is best not to add this herb to your protocol unless under the supervision of a skilled practitioner.

After adding Green Chiretta to my core protocol, I did experience a mild Herxheimer reaction. I suffered from nausea and discomfort in my abdomen, accompanied by a bout of diarrhea which lasted for a couple of days. Once the spate of diarrhea ended, I continued taking the Green Chiretta without any further discomfort. By understanding what the herb does and knowing ahead of time that a Herxheimer reaction could occur, I actually welcomed the discomfort. It provided proof that more bacteria were dying off and that thought was extremely satisfying.

To boost my dilapidated immune system and support the loss and restructure of collagen, I added the following supplements to my daily protocol (specific dosages can be found in the Appendix): selenium, cat's claw, Siberian ginseng, astragalus, vitamin C, a vitamin B complex, vitamin E, echinacea *angustifolia*, royal jelly, zinc, and copper. You are right if you think that my kitchen shelves looked like a witch's closet.

After about six months, I had regained considerable strength and was beginning to feel much better. I slowly let the immune system and collagen supplements run out, but stayed on the core protocol including the Green Chiretta.

Spirochetes are clever organisms. They learn to hide and morph into different forms when things become uncomfortable in their home––our cells. When transformed and encapsulated, they can remain in that state for up to two years (!) before they absolutely must feed again. I suspected that through the massive attack on their existence by my daily regimen of supplements, the bacteria were cleverly encapsulated, awaiting better times. But time was running out for them. Ha!

In order to be one hundred percent sure that the bacteria did not have a chance to feed and multiply once they reemerged from their encapsulated state, I decided to stay on the core protocol for a full two years. I figured that, over the two-year span, my immune system would have a chance to recuperate fully and sharpen its weapons. When after their hibernation the spirochetes were on the go again, they would be in serious peril.

To rid myself of the bacteria and to boost my immune system further, I also engaged in other activities that I knew would be helpful. Our hunter-gatherer forebears understood the importance of sweat lodges and steam bathing. The tradition of healing through sweating has been carried forward through the ages and used by various different cultures. Inhabitants of the Caribbean Islands have long been experts at curing spirochete infections by the use of sweat baths. They understood that heat (an induced fever) kills bacteria. The *Borrelia* bacterium thrives at 96.8°F (36°C). It loves the human body. But at a temperature of 107.6°F (42°C) it dies off. I began taking regular saunas, sweating and deeply breathing in air heated to temperatures of up to 180°F followed by refreshing dips in cold water pools. The thought of "frying" these unwanted tenants in my body while sweating gave me great pleasure and made these regular sauna dates an enjoyable treat.

The islanders also prescribed strenuous physical labor to assist the healing process of the body. I learned that the rigorous use of muscle tissue, pressure on bones and other body parts, accompanied by sweating, would increase blood circulation and oxygen flow and assist in the healing. Physical labor was hard in the beginning for me, as weakness from the illness was overwhelming. But with each month I gained strength, the physical work becoming more and more enjoyable.

✳

As I conclude this personal account, it has been two years and six months since I first got infected by Lyme bacteria. I am overjoyed to report that all my symptoms have disappeared. My strength and stamina are back.

Today––every single day––I am amazed at what my body is capable of doing. I am especially grateful for the clarity of mind and the ability to function normally again––maybe in some ways even better than before. Should you be infected with Lyme disease, I wish you from the bottom of my heart the same success. And I hope very much that this book may assist you along your recovery.

PART II

TICKS AND LYME SPIROCHETES

"In order to change
we must be sick and tired of being sick and tired."

—unknown

When I began my research about Lyme disease, I had no idea what interesting information I would find. I started out in desperate search for an alternative treatment for Lyme disease: antibiotics had failed me, and I was ill and miserable. Ticks and bacteria were the last thing on my mind. What I discovered about ticks and bacteria, however, was beyond fascinating. Both became an integral part of my journey.

Ticks are by no means my favorite creatures. But how they have survived and continue to do so in our ever-changing environment is intriguing. While many animals tend to lean toward or become subject to extinction, ticks belong to that group of species that not only survives nicely but seems to evolve and get stronger with each generation. New kinds of ticks are being discovered all the time, and with them, unfortunately for us, new types of harmful bacteria as well.

And then there are the bacteria, the underlying cause of Lyme disease. Having been around for millions of years, they know how to maneuver, adapt, and survive. What I learned about these microorganisms left me speechless. It is beyond science fiction. Through my research, I could not help but go from absolutely despising them to, ultimately, admiring them. We would benefit tremendously could we just understand how these organisms exist, adapt, and evolve.

If you are looking for treatments, skip this chapter and go straight to Part III, Treatments. But if you have the time to read about ticks and bacteria, I highly recommend you do so. Knowing and understanding them will help tremendously in your recovery. Plus, you may be amazed at what you will discover.

TICKS

"As I see it, every day you do one of two things:
build health or produce disease in yourself."

--Adelle Davis

Nobody likes ticks. Actually, that's not exactly true. During my research I did meet some people who do like ticks-- enough to study them exclusively. Not me. I don't like them, thank you very much. But learning about ticks in relation to Lyme disease was very helpful and an eye opener.

We don't like ticks because they are parasites that carry harmful bacteria. They are carriers of *Borrelia burgdorferi*, the bacteria that causes Lyme disease. Ticks serve as ideal vehicles for these bacteria. To our dismay, these small and often infected creatures bite us in search for a blood meal and so transmit the bacteria to us. Humans have become an increasingly favored host for ticks. We are simply a source of food to them, though this has not always been the case. In the past, they have had many other hosts to satisfy their need for a blood meal. But considering the changes our world has gone through (and continues to go through), that humans have become a readily available host for ticks is no coincidence.

At one time, and not that long ago in our extensive history, massive bison herds which included millions of animals roamed the Great Plains. At the same time, other animals--elk, deer, and antelopes driven by the changes of the seasons--migrated from east to west. These herds were a primary food source for ticks. With the help of these herds, ticks--unable to move far on their own--were able to hitchhike enormous distances while enjoying a protein-rich blood meal. But through the changes of the land and the eradication of much if not all of these animal herds, massive ecological and biological shifts took place.

These transformations altered not only animal populations on the surface of the earth, but in the air as well. History documents enormous, nowadays unimaginable, flocks of birds––stories that sound like fairy tales to us today. These flocks were indeed so enormous that when the birds migrated, skies would be darkened for several days. We have lost these feathery friends forever, but we have lost more than the birds themselves. These now-extinct creatures once consumed massive amounts of insects, including ticks and tick eggs. They also served as hosts for bacteria.

Before ticks feed on large mammals, they seek rodents and other small animals for their first blood meal. It is through these rodents, actually, that the ticks become infected themselves, as small rodents are the main bacterial carriers.

Rodents are also a major food source for foxes, wolves, coyote, and other four-footed carnivores, as well as raptors. A continuous decline of carnivores and raptors allows for the increase of the rodent population. Without the carnivores who keep their population at bay, rodents enjoy free rein to prosper and multiply, creating an imbalance in nature. More rodents equals more hosts for bacteria.

Ticks lay a large number of eggs. Luckily, not all of them manage to molt into their next stage, because insect predators feed on them. The abundant use of pesticides has dramatically reduced the number of these so-called "unwanted" insects. What those who use pesticides may not consider is that these unwanted insects also feed on tick eggs and larvae. And that the absence of these insects allows for more eggs to hatch and for more ticks to grow and multiply.

These significant changes in the environment have forced ticks to adapt. Through the reduction and extinction of many animals, ticks lost millions of readily available hosts. Without those massive herds, they were forced to look for food elsewhere. This was not a threat to their survival, as other animals quickly moved into the vast spaces where herds used to roam.

Ticks are highly evolved species. Driven by their survival instinct, they adapted quickly. Faced with the lack of large mammals, they simply jumped species. Ticks went from feeding on buffalo, elk, and antelopes to feeding on small mammals, deer, and moose, which became readily available. And they discovered another food source—humans. More and more humans filled the void, living in the areas once occupied by large mammals. We have become a source of nourishment for ticks.

Nature is splendid. Had we not messed with it and driven these animals into extinction, things might be in much better harmony today. Bacteria and ticks might still be busy messing around with animals instead of humans.

Ticks are the primary carrier of *Borrelia burgdorferi*. They are parasites with an unusual life cycle. During their lifetime, they experience three major stages.

The adult female lays approximately two to three thousand eggs in the spring. In late summer or early fall, larvae hatch from these eggs. The larvae are bacteria-free, as the mother tick does not pass on bacteria to its offspring. This is actually a good thing for us, as the larva is small, barely the size of the prick of a needle; we would hardly be able to detect this tan-colored dot, were it to feed on us. If a larva were to attach to us, it would feed, get engorged, drop off, and be on its way without causing any harm. At least we do not have to worry about getting sick from a larva bite.

Eager to grow and molt into a new stage, the larva's single purpose is to feed. If it cannot feed, it will die: if the weather gets too cold before it has a chance to find a meal, it will not be able to survive. It knows that getting food is crucial for survival, and it needs to find it quickly.

Blood from other animals is the only item on the ticks' menu. Like bloodsucking arthropods such as mosquitoes and fleas, ticks need blood. At all stages of life, they need it specifically to be able to molt into their next stage and ultimately produce eggs and multiply. Ticks are essentially bloodsucking parasites.

Larvae are unable to travel far for a meal. Lazily, they crawl up a stem of grass and wait until a small mammal passes by. This would typically be a mouse (a white-footed, not a house mouse), a chipmunk, or a shrew. Small rodents not only deliver a tasty blood meal to the larvae but are the primary host for *Borrelia burgdorferi* bacteria. About 90 percent of the rodent population in the United States is infected with this bacterium.

Once a blood meal has been consumed by the larva, it has most likely become infected. Satisfied and fully engorged, it drops off its host and begins its first molting process during the following winter.

Come spring, the larva has molted into a bacterium-carrying nymph. And it is hungry. It will immediately set out to "quest" ––the entomological term for the tick's behavior when finding a host to feed on. A nymph is slightly larger than a larva and can attach to a human. Typically, however, it will seek small mammals––foxes, raccoons, ground-dwelling birds, even lizards if available. After three to six days of feeding, now fully engorged, it will drop once more and, during the summer months, begin the molting process into an adult tick. Most Lyme disease cases in humans are caused by nymphs.

By fall, the nymph has grown into an adult tick. Its shape and its purpose have slightly changed. It is now larger and easily detectable. If it is male, it will not feed again. The male's sole role is to find a female and to mate. Instinctively, it will hitch a ride on a large mammal like a deer or a moose. Once on the host, it will wander around until it finds a female, mate, and then die off. A male tick can only transfer bacteria in its state as a nymph.

The female on the other hand experiences the urge to feed in order to produce eggs. Adult female ticks will look for a host of significant size to get a rich blood meal and to remain undetected. This host is referred to as the "reproductive host," because the female tick needs to get enough protein-rich blood to produce her eggs. She will feed on any mammal she can find—skunks, raccoons, opossums, turkeys, squirrels, chipmunks, deer, moose.

After selecting her host, the adult female will wander around, looking for an ideal place to latch on. Female ticks are picky and follow an internal instinct to look for a safe place. They like areas that guarantee them protection from being groomed off or eaten. They prefer dampness, moisture, darkness, and warmth. In humans they favor the armpits, the crotch area, the beginning of the hair line, or facial hair. They take their time to find this ideal spot and can wander around for an entire day. Once the tick has found what it is looking for, it will latch on to its host and feed for three to six days, depending on the size of the host. In humans, a tick will feed three to four days before it is fully engorged and drops off. An adult tick can increase in size one hundred times while feeding.

Satisfied, and having acquired the protein necessary, the female drops off its host and overwinters. Not until the following spring will it lay two to three thousand eggs and then die off as well. And so, the life circle of the tick has been completed. Luckily, not all of the tick eggs will survive. Many insects and birds will feed on them before they have a chance to molt into larvae.

A tick has a typical life cycle of two years in which it overwinters twice. Most of this time is spent off the host, molting into its next life stage, looking for a new host, or hibernating in leaf litter. If the adult tick is unsuccessful in finding a host in the fall, it can overwinter and search again in the spring. This is the reason why we find, in addition to nymphs, adult ticks during springtime. Recent studies show that ticks have learned to survive even multiple winters if no hosts are available. Dang!

Normally, ticks feed only once—a single blood meal—at each stage of their life. This means two meals for a male tick and three meals for a female tick over the course of their existence. However, if circumstances require, a tick can feed in stages as well. A partially fed tick that has been groomed off a host can reattach to another host. In this case, bacteria can be transmitted very quickly to the new host. But more about bacteria later.

Hosts

Hosts are critical for the survival of ticks, but also influence the ticks' infection rate. Hosts have one major purpose for ticks––to serve as a food source. Unfortunately, hosts most often are bacterial reservoirs as well and hence pass pathogens on to ticks during feeding.

Hosts come in all sizes. Larvae feed on the smallest hosts, like mice and shrews, while nymphs attach to larger mammals, including pets and small farm animals. Adult ticks need large animals––deer, moose, and others––for a richer protein meal. In areas where there are no large mammals available, however, such as on islands, nymphs and adult ticks have cleverly adapted. They are thriving and multiplying quite nicely by feeding on nothing but small animals while passing pathogens back and forth.

Humans can be bitten by ticks of all ticks' life stages–– larvae to adult. As previously mentioned, most common infections in humans result from nymph bites.

The availability of hosts greatly influences the number of ticks in a given area. If more white-footed mice are present, a higher chance of survival for larvae and nymphs is guaranteed. The same is true for deer. A large presence of deer––another favorite host––in an area pretty much guarantees a large number of ticks, as deer serve as an excellent source of a high-protein meal for nymphs and adult ticks.

Not all hosts present equal opportunity for ticks. The "success rate" of ticks feeding on white-footed mice and white-tailed deer is nearly 50 percent. By comparison, the success rate of ticks feeding on chipmunks, shrews, squirrels, or ground birds drops to less than 25 percent. Clever as they are, ticks have learned over time which hosts serve them best. And they have adapted well to changes in the availability of host populations. Ticks know that choosing the right host will affect their ability to survive, molt, and lay eggs. They purposefully choose hosts with a high rate of feeding success.

The ability for a tick to survive while on a host depends largely on the grooming habits of the host—and some hosts are very good groomers. Opossums are excellent groomers. Only 4 percent of ticks succeed in feeding on opossums. When opossums waddle around at night, they pick up dozens of ticks which they will meticulously groom off their coat and swallow. Scientists have estimated that opossums consume as many as five thousand ticks per season. Cats, like the opossum, spend much time grooming and eating ticks that have latched on. Some animals, such as moose, groom very little or not at all. (Eating the ticks, by the way, will not infect cats or other groomers.)

How many ticks are infected by *Borrelia burgdorferi* depends also on how competent the host community is in serving as a reservoir; if hosts are not very good at maintaining the bacteria, there will be fewer infected ticks in that area. Some wild mice have developed a particular gene variant that makes them immune to the *Borrelia burgdorferi* bacteria. This has led to experimentation with genetically modified mice. Scientists are introducing these mice into contained environments such as islands to observe their development around infected ticks. It is to be expected, however, that the increasing resistance of these mice to the bacteria will trigger an adaptation in the bacteria as well. The evolutionary race between host and bacteria continues.

All hosts react differently to *Borrelia burgdorferi*. The reaction to the bacteria depends on the host's immune system and other factors, such as grooming habits and genetic makeup. Dogs and humans get quite sick from the *Borrelia burgdorferi* bacteria. On the other hand, mice, shrews, and chipmunks can be infected and show very few symptoms. A white-footed mouse that is infected with the bacteria in a laboratory shows no difference in behavior or wellbeing in comparison to a noninfected mouse.

If we could just understand what the immune system of a white-footed mouse knows, maybe we could implement that knowhow into the human fabric. Who would have thought that we could learn something so important from a mouse?

CLIMATE AND ENVIRONMENT

Climate plays an important role in the survival of ticks. Contrary to common belief, ticks thrive well in the cold, surviving temperatures as low as minus 30 degrees Celsius (minus 22 degrees Fahrenheit). They actually live twice as long in colder climates. But essentially, if the tick has a choice where to reside, it favors warmer surroundings.

While the world may be frozen on the surface, the tick patiently waits underneath the snow, comfortably tucked into leaf litter until temperatures rise above 40 degrees F. At that temperature, or warmer, it is motivated to crawl to the surface and begin its questing. Adult ticks are tougher and can quest at a lower temperature than nymphs. If the temperature remains unusually cold during spring or summer, ticks are not able to develop fully and are forced to slow down their life cycle. Therefore, our increasing warmer growing seasons may affect the tick population more positively than warmer winters do.

Over the past decades, heat has increased in our cities as well. What were once considered Lyme-disease-safe environments have become hot spots for ticks. City parks, cemeteries, and areas with greenery offer an ideal and comfortable residence for ticks. Hosts are readily available as well, fluttering in to settle in trees or strolling in and out of these places on the ground. Ticks can find a meal on ground-feeding birds and small mammals, like mice, and unfortunately, they do not restrain themselves from latching on to our pets––when we take doggy for a walk in the park––or to us and our children during playtime.

Higher elevations typically have colder climates. In previous studies, ticks have been found in large numbers at elevations of up to five hundred feet. Their numbers dropped drastically and fell to almost zero at an elevation of one thousand feet and higher. With ongoing climate change, however, ticks are able to find warmer temperatures in higher elevations and continue to move into areas which were previously of little interest to them.

The change in climate also affects the host population. A hard winter will knock back the population of white-footed mice, which will result in fewer available hosts and hence fewer ticks the following year. On the other hand, a year where we have a larger number of acorns than usual—a favorite food source for mice—is typically followed by a year with a greater number of mice. The presence of these mice in plentiful numbers assures food, survival, and procreation for ticks, and we will see a larger number of ticks the following year.

If there are lots of foxes and coyotes in an area, chances are that we have fewer ticks. Foxes and coyotes feed primarily on mice and greatly help to knock down the mice population. The same is true for raptors. Changes in surrounding woodlands and forests, as we see in developing areas everywhere, directly affect the number and type of hosts. These changes in turn influence the number of ticks present in that area. Any factor that influences the host community has a direct effect on the density and infection rate of ticks.

Ticks need moisture to survive. Humidity is a big deal for ticks. Should the leaf litter dry out completely, they will die. This is the reason why we see fewer ticks during a dry summer or in areas with dry climates. If it is too moist, on the other hand, ticks will develop a fungal infection—at last, good news for a rainy summer. Ticks are smart, however, and will pick places with mild temperatures and relatively high humidity, if they have a choice. But they are essentially quite lazy. They are incapable of moving far and prefer to hitchhike wherever their host takes them.

If temperature and humidity allow, they will begin to quest, crawling up a stem of grass and patiently waiting until a mammal passes by. If unsuccessful, the tick begins to dehydrate and has to return below the leaf litter to hydrate. It will quest less in dry air than in moist air. This is why we see more ticks in the spring, a generally wet time of the year, than in late summer, when it has not rained for a while. Dry surroundings are a serious threat for the survival of ticks.

Ticks are plentiful in their ideal environment. New England with its moist climate, its many trees and consequential leaf litter, is such an ideal environment. To collect tick specimens in early spring, researchers in Vermont have dragged a cloth the size of one yard by four yards through grass. In an area of approximately twenty yards, as many as four hundred ticks have been found attached to the cloth. Yikes!

✳

All of New England, but especially Vermont, has experienced a dramatic increase in Lyme disease over the past ten years. In the 90s and early 2000s, very few cases of Lyme disease in the United States were reported to the Center of Disease Control (CDC). The CDC now receives reports of thirty thousand cases of Lyme disease per year nationwide. However, the CDC's numbers are highly underrepresented due to the notorious misdiagnosis of the disease. According to the CDC, the currently reported number of cases would have to be multiplied by at least ten (three hundred thousand cases a year) to reach an accurate count! This increase is partially due to the movement of ticks which carry and spread the bacteria, as well as an increase in the awareness about Lyme disease by practitioners and the general public. Over the course of the past three years, Vermont has become the state with the second-highest rate of reported Lyme disease incidences. (As of this writing, Maine has the highest reported number of cases.)

Types of Ticks

With the northward expansion of the **blacklegged tick** (also referred to simply as the deer tick) we notice a simultaneous northward expansion of Lyme disease. This particular tick––the blacklegged (deer) tick––is the primary, but not the only carrier of *Borrelia burgdorferi* among ticks.

There are currently thirteen tick species that we are aware of in New England. Most of these ticks are quite rare and only five of the thirteen species are actually known to bite humans. Of the five tick species that do bite humans, four can transmit diseases.

Of the sixteen known tick-borne diseases in the United States transmitted by ticks to humans, there are mainly four that occur in New England. These four diseases are, 99 percent of the time, transmitted by the blacklegged (deer) tick. The most common is Lyme disease.

However, the other three very serious tick-borne diseases transmitted by the blacklegged (deer) tick are on the rise. Before 2011, we experienced fewer than ten cases of anaplasmosis per year in Vermont. By 2016, this number had increased to two hundred cases per year and continues to be on the rise. Vermont is now the state with the highest incidence of anaplasmosis in the country––a hot spot.

More and more cases of Powassan (POW) virus disease and babesiosis, a microscopic parasite that infects red blood cells, are being reported in Vermont. These diseases are also transmitted by the blacklegged (deer) tick and are very serious illnesses. Over one third of the cases result in hospitalization for respiratory support, intravenous fluids, or medications necessary to reduce swelling in the brain. For older patients, or patients suffering from an already compromised immune system, an infection by these bacteria or viruses have rarely but occasionally resulted in death.

Unfortunately, it is very difficult to differentiate between the individual tick-borne diseases, as all tick-borne infections have similar symptoms. A typical symptom in response to a tick bite is a bullseye rash in about thirty percent of cases. This is the only positive and definite indicator of an infection caused by a tick bite. Other symptoms include flulike symptoms, headache, neck stiffness, muscle and joint pain, fever of various degrees, soreness, tiredness, body rash, nausea, weakness, and in some cases paralysis.

The **American dog tick** (also called wood tick) is common and bigger than the blacklegged deer tick. It is good to know the difference between blacklegged (deer) ticks and American dog ticks. Besides adult American dog ticks being larger than blacklegged (deer) ticks, American dog ticks have characteristic white markings on their back. And, unlike the blacklegged (deer) tick, this tick has brown legs. The American dog tick is not thought to transmit Lyme disease, but it can, although rarely, transmit other diseases to humans.

The lone star tick is mostly seen in Southern states. But it is slowly making its way north as well. It is still rare, however. As the name suggests, this tick is easily recognizable as it has a star on its back.

The lone star tick spreads the bacteria *ehrlichia* causing ehrlichiosis. It can also cause an allergy to red meat. When the lone star tick feeds on a deer, in some incidences a microscopic amount of deer blood infiltrates into the tick. When the tick later in its life happens to feed on a human, traces of deer blood can enter the human blood stream. This can cause an allergic reaction from the immune system, triggered by the presence of deer blood protein in the blood stream. The allergic reaction is different from a bacterial or viral infection and over time should recede on its own. By the way, meat lovers, do not fear. You cannot get this allergy by eating venison from an infected animal. The red-meat allergy only happens if deer blood is directly introduced into the human blood stream.

The **winter tick** poses very little threat to humans. It prefers to feed mainly on large mammals. This tick is different from its cousins, as it remains on the same host throughout all its life stages.

The winter tick will cause anemia, skin irritation, and hair loss on animals. If enough winter ticks are attached to a single host, and feed and reproduce on that animal, they can even cause the death of the host. Moose do not groom. Since winter ticks prefer to feed on them, these ticks are particularly harmful to this group of animals.

Like the blacklegged (deer) tick, the winter tick prefers to feed on deer as well. With more deer in an area, a higher number of winter ticks is guaranteed. And the higher the number of winter ticks, the greater the threat will be to the survival of the local moose population. This is just another eye-opening example of the interconnectedness in nature.

Nature is constantly changing and evolving. These changes, unfortunately for us, include the migration and appearance of new tick species.

The **longhorn tick** is native to China, Korea, and Japan and established in New Zealand and Australia. It was not known to be established in the United States until November 2017. Preferring a moist climate, it has taken residence on the east coast.

Longhorn ticks are small, reddish-brown ticks without any distinctive markings. They feed on wildlife and livestock but also on cats, dogs, and humans. So far, they have not been associated with diseases in the United States, but have been the cause for a number of animal and human diseases in Asia and Australia.

Like the discovery of the longhorn tick, unknown tick species, as well as ticks so far known to reside only in foreign countries, are now being discovered in the United States. It is an ongoing challenge for our scientists to keep up with the rapid changes in the lives of ticks, to understand what known and unknown bacteria they carry, where these ticks reside, and where they hitchhike to and from.

Tick Removal

Once a tick has latched on and is imbedded, it will take quite a bit of force to remove it successfully. The tick is an evolved species and has learned over time what works for its survival. It knows that if it does not latch on securely, it will most likely be groomed off and possibly eaten. Therefore, to resist grooming, it buries its entire head into the skin of its host to feed. A luffa sponge or washcloth will not remove an embedded tick, no matter how small or large the tick is.

People have experimented with tick-removal ever since these critters began latching on to pets and humans. It is important to remove the entire tick, especially the embedded head. Most commonly, tweezers or plastic tick removal gadgets are used for the task. Gadgets specifically made for pets will work just as well for humans. In either case, it is crucial to tug gently on the tick's body and not to twist, so the head will not break off––even without the body attached, the head is still transmissive. It is also important to apply only gentle pressure with tweezers. If too much pressure is applied, the tick will regurgitate its stomach contents––including bacteria, if infected––and transmit it to the host before letting go. It is best to have either tweezers or an actual tick removal gadget in your backpack and your home apothecary at all times.

TICKS AND LYME-CONTROL STRATEGIES

There are various strategies that can help to control the population of ticks. Substances such as acaricides, which are pesticides, are used both in medicine and agriculture to kill ticks and mites without harming the host. New types of acaricides have been developed to specifically target mice and deer. The idea is that the animals come in contact with the substance and then, with a little help, spread it among their young––for mice, with the help of cotton balls and bait boxes, and for deer, with a four-poster structure near a feeding point. As you can imagine, it would be hard as an individual to successfully target all the small mammals and deer in a large area. As a community, however, these measures are more promising.

A reduction of available hosts themselves would translate into an immediate effect on the tick population. Deer culling or fencing limit the range of these large hosts and therefore the spread of the bacteria. On islands, entire deer populations have been eliminated in attempts to reduce the number of ticks.

There are ways for individuals to successfully reduce the tick population around a homestead. Leaf litter and brush piles in the yard, as well as leaves on wood piles and stone walls, should be removed. The less moisture, which ticks need to molt, the fewer ticks will be present. Keeping the lawn maintained and short will help dry the grass and the earth below and so reduce moisture. Pruning trees and bushes allows sunlight to penetrate to the ground and help dry it out. A border of stone or dry mulch between a wooded area and a lawn will keep ticks from moving out of the woods and onto the lawn. Bird feeders should be placed beyond the stone or dry mulch barrier. If walking trails in the woods are kept wide and open, deer and other mammals will be discouraged from roaming there.

Unfortunately, as of this writing, there are no human vaccines to prevent Lyme disease. A previously available vaccine caused debilitating side effects and had to be pulled off the market. There are, however, medications for our pets. Once ingested, the medication circulates in the bloodstream of the animal. If a tick bites the medicated animal, the blood tastes bad, and the tick will let go of its host and look elsewhere for a tastier meal.

Other measures, such as biocontrol, look promising. Experiments have been done with parasitic wasps, nematodes (worms), and fungi, where the soil-inhabiting fungus Metarhizium seems most promising.

Another fun and useful biocontrol method is the keeping of Guinea hens. They are busy all day long grooming your backyard or lawn for insects, including ticks. And as a bonus, they deliver an egg for breakfast.

Wearing light-colored clothes helps you to detect ticks that might latch on as you stroll through fields or woods. Ticks are clever and tend to hide in seams. An easy and certain way to rid clothes of any ticks is to put them into the dryer for half an hour. The heat will kill all ticks and any living bacteria, if the tick was infected.

Challenged by this rapidly growing epidemic, the scientific community is working hard on developing solutions. Genetically modified and bacteria-resistant animals are one approach to conquer the epidemic. Developing vaccines for mice, deer, and humans is another way we may gain protection against Lyme disease, at least temporarily.

It is also an ongoing race between the accelerated adaptation of clever bacteria and any defensive measures our immune system is capable of, or may be able to develop. The ultimate goal would be to change our genetic makeup, so we too become resistant to the Lyme bacteria by developing a gene variant similar to what some mice have managed to do. A lofty goal indeed.

LYME SPIROCHETES: BORRELIA BURGDORFERI

"Every patient carries her or his own doctor inside."

--Albert Schweitzer

My research relied upon many sources. Much of what is detailed in this particular chapter, I owe to Stephen Harrod Buhner and his extensive work on Lyme disease, which he documented in several volumes. Should you be interested in knowing and understanding everything there is to know about Lyme disease--including details and recent discoveries about *Borrelia burgdorferi*--and if you have the time to devote to this impressive volume, you would do well to read Buhner's bestselling book *Healing Lyme*.

The bacterium *Borrelia burgdorferi*--the Lyme spirochete--is the actual culprit causing Lyme disease. *Borrelia burgdorferi* may well be the most intelligent and creative microorganisms that we know of. They have accumulated an impressive bank of know-how and developed thousands of ways to express themselves. Science fiction in its wildest dreams could not make up what these bacteria are capable of.

After evolving for billions of years, *Borrelia burgdorferi* bacteria have had ample time to develop clever and stealthy ways to adapt to changes in the environment. They endured extreme upheavals during the course of the earth's evolution, and then, three million to as recent as twelve thousand years ago, they managed to survive quite nicely among the glaciers that covered the earth at the time.

We estimate that humans have been around for two to three hundred thousand, possibly several million years. Still, we are a relatively young species in comparison to other life forms, which scientists speculate began some three billion years ago. This makes us and our bacteria-fighting immune system relatively inexperienced compared to these ancient organisms.

While human beings are increasing in number with mind-boggling speed, other species are becoming extinct at a rapid rate. But bacteria with eons of life experience are not bothered much by the comings and goings of one or another species. The survival of these microorganisms is under no threat, and their presence does not seem to decline. As their surroundings change, they merely shift from one vehicle to the next to ensure survival. Bacteria seek whatever convenient host they can find. It is only natural that, with the massive increase of the human population and the decrease in many animal species, humans have become a preferred and readily available host.

We generally think of the tick as the sole host for *Borrelia burgdorferi*. Bacteria, however, were aware that in order to survive they needed to establish themselves in more than just one species and in more than just one place. Ever so successful at their game, they have been found all over the world, including among penguins in the inhospitable climate of the South Pole. There are no longer any Lyme-bacteria-free zones on our planet. Every state in the United States has documented cases of Lyme disease.

Birds, as one example, are fabulous carriers of Lyme spirochetes, continually spreading them across the globe and ultimately depositing them around bird feeders. From there, the spirochetes are picked up and spread locally by other animals. In recent research, among North American birds every songbird tested turned out to be a carrier for the bacteria. Furthermore, researchers detected spirochetes in mosquitoes, mites, fleas, lizards, and biting flies. The bacteria were also found in the feces of infected animals, cleverly packaged as borrelial biofilms. (More about biofilms later.)

Originally, we thought we had to be concerned with mice and deer as main reservoirs for these bacteria. In fact, all small ground-based mammals are now reservoirs for spirochetes. Farm animals, dogs, rabbits, raccoons, horses, and other large animals have also been shown to carry the bacteria. All in all, over three hundred different species of mammals, birds, and reptiles are spirochete carriers.

Once transmitted to a host, spirochetes don't necessarily stay there forever. If they choose to, they can spread with ease from one host to the next. They pick the precise real estate––the place where they will make their new home within a host––according to their intention. They either bury themselves deeply into tissue, if they desire to stay, or they colonize in an area where a quicker transfer to a new host is guaranteed. For quick transfer, the bladder is a perfect place to colonize. When peed out, now securely packaged within a biofilm (more about biofilms later), the bacteria find themselves in a temporary residence––lush grasses perhaps––until another animal comes along and ingests the spirochetes.

For humans, the situation is not much brighter. Once they have infected a human, Lyme spirochetes are transmitted by humans to humans through bodily fluids–– specifically semen, vaginal secretion, tears, and breast milk. Even a fetus is not safe if the mother is infected.

Spirochetes are wormlike and superintelligent bacteria. They have learned to cope with all sorts of unpleasant circumstances and have come up with many remarkable schemes to avert them. When out of nourishment, or attacked by the immune response of the host, or threatened by antibiotics, the bacterium simply changes from its wormlike shape into an encysted form. Here it can hibernate nicely, not unlike the seed of a plant, for up to three years, until the danger has passed or food has become available again. They also don't mind if it gets a little cold. Encysted spirochetes that have survived freezing and thawing are still capable of infecting their host.

Spirochetes have two motors, one in the front and one in the back, and a wiggling tail. These allow them to burrow themselves deeply into tissue, places where the immune system and its army of antibodies have a hard time finding and fighting them, such as collagen in joints. The Lyme disease spirochetes are the fastest burrowers of all known spirochetes.

Choosing ticks as their primary vehicle is not coincidental. Lyme spirochetes are an extremely intelligent microorganism and have established the perfect setup for their survival. As we have learned, an immature tick must feed on small rodents to grow from a larval into a nymphal tick. While feeding on a rodent or other small ground-based mammal, the larva picks up a side dish of spirochetes. In nine out of ten cases, a tick will become infected if its host carries the bacteria. Later, when the tick has matured to an adult state and prefers to feed on a larger mammal, it passes the bacteria on to a larger host.

Because ticks need to feed on various hosts throughout their life cycles, bacteria that have taken residence in ticks are assured a thorough spread across many hosts. This aids in the bacteria's survival and contributes to their ever-growing databank of immune system information.

Over the course of their existence, ticks and spirochetes have developed a good relationship. Ticks are hungry and need to feed to survive and reproduce, which works well for spirochetes. Ticks are also highly evolved species and know how to go about their business.

The ticks' particular way to obtain a blood meal, is a perfect scenario for spirochetes to transfer to a new host. To ensure a stealth attack and ample time to feed, the tick's saliva, a potent anesthetic, shuts down parts of the immune response of the host during a bite. Without a proper immune response, it is much easier for the tick to feed for the two to three days necessary to get fully engorged. This fabulous setup gives the spirochetes plenty of time to study and ultimately enter the new host undetected.

Some spirochetes already present in the tick's saliva and gut will transfer immediately once the tick has sawed through the skin of its host. The rapid transfer assures survival for the bacteria––get there while you can––and once inside their new host, some of those first-comers will instantly change form to remain undetected.

The majority of spirochetes, however, wait patiently for the blood meal to arrive in the tick's midgut. Once the blood of the host is analyzed, they take the cue, rapidly adapting to their new host and changing their DNA if necessary. Lyme bacteria are considered to be the most complex bacteria of them all. They possess twenty-four extra DNA segments which they are constantly rearranging, depending on the characteristics and the environment of their host. They have the largest number of DNA replications among any known bacteria. This allows them to adjust with ease to an immune response or other attack such as antibiotics once the bacteria have arrived in the host.

Having adapted to their new host, the spirochetes multiply to triple or even quadruple their number while still in the tick's gut. The impressive artillery then marches to the tick's salivary glands where the bacteria begin a back-and-forth conversation. This conversation is so intricate and sophisticated, it not only focuses on the type of host that the tick has attached to and the precise details of the host's immune system, but even includes the climate of the host's environment.

Spirochetes have learned how to interpret an unbelievable number of characteristics of the many hosts available to them. Each infection challenges the bacteria to adapt in order to take residence and thrive. Since every bodily ecosystem and each immune system is different from host to host, spirochetes expand their knowhow with every new infection. The host's information is quickly added to the bacteria's databank. And so, the spirochete's incredible accumulation of data continues to expand. In response to this highly sophisticated information, the bacteria alter their genetic structure and if necessary, their behavior. The spirochetes *Borrelia burgdorferi* are experts at these adaptations. They do so in not just one way, but create several versions of themselves to ensure survivability. This guarantees that they are able to remain undetected. Through this strategy, spirochetes actually create new versions of themselves with each invasion! Did I mention science fiction?

This ability to adapt to their new environment by changing their DNA and their shape causes infections that are literally unique in each host. Because of the uniqueness of the infections, the characteristics and symptoms of Lyme disease change over and over again. In addition, an infected host may carry various different types of Lyme bacteria. Some of these strains have evolved to a degree that they are not at all susceptible to the efforts of our immune systems or to treatments with antibiotics.

Spirochetes are very thin and grow extremely slowly. This makes them difficult to study in a laboratory. (Personally, I think that's just another scheme they have developed to outsmart us.) Hence, to this day, very little is known about them. Their cousin, the syphilis bacteria, which we have studied for almost a century, still cannot be grown in a laboratory.

Ticks are parasites and so are spirochetes. They cannot live without harvesting from a host. Unlike ticks, who prefer a meal of blood, spirochetes have a preference for collagenous tissue, which is found throughout the body. Wherever the bacteria take residence and feed, we notice symptoms.

First, at the initial infection, the symptoms are flulike, with a bullseye rash in about 30 percent of infections. The bullseye rash is the only definite marker for a Lyme disease diagnosis. The red rash of the bullseye indicates an immune system's efforts to fight the invader. If the bacteria succeed in sidestepping the immune system's attempt to kill them off, they continue to make their way ever deeper into the body.

The bacteria have learned, not only to hide from an immune response, but the best places to hide in the host. There, in the hard-to-detect places of a body, they cleverly reduce their activity, giving the impression that the infection has resolved or treatment has been successful. Consequently, the immune system calms down and the attack on the invader is greatly reduced. When all is safe again in the surroundings of their hiding place, the bacteria quickly multiply. This time, however, having had plenty of time to study the characteristics of the attacker, they regrow themselves as an immune-resistant subpopulation. Holy cow!

The hide-and-seek game between the immune system and the ever-changing bacteria is the beginning of the chronic phase of Lyme disease. We may experience arthritis if they have rooted themselves in the joints; various skin manifestations, if they are rooted in the collagen under the skin; heart disease if they have found their way to the heart; or neurological problems, once they have made their way through the blood-brain barrier.

After their successful siege, and after having taken residence in their preferred location in the host, the bacteria feed. They use substances––among them their feces––to break down tissue. These tissues could be myelin sheaths in the brain, cartilage in joints, or ligaments. Just about everywhere where our bodies have collagen. Once the tissue has become a tasty soup of nutrients, the spirochetes sit down to a hearty meal. They literally eat us from the inside out.

In the course of the breakdown of tissue, many additional medical complications ensue. For example, once the brain is lacking the sheaths that protect the nerves, the nerves begin to malfunction. Furthermore, during the breakdown of the myelin sheaths, the bacteria set free a myelin protein and release it into places in the brain where it does not belong. The alarmed immune system attempts to remove these substances. Eventually the immune system considers the myelin proteins, which are still in their proper place, as foreign substances as well; it attacks them and causes even further neural damage.

It is not until recently that we have come to understand the correlation between chronic infections caused by spirochetes in the brain and central nervous system, and diseases whose origin we do not understand. Lyme disease sufferers have been misdiagnosed with illnesses such as multiple sclerosis, Parkinson's disease, Alzheimer's disease, dementia, even bipolar disorder and schizophrenia. Recent studies of deceased Alzheimer's patients showed that 90 percent were hosting spirochetes!

Luckily, there are remedies that can reverse the damage, including damage to neural structures in the brain caused by these destructive invaders. We will talk about these remedies in Part III, Treatments.

Spirochetes have more tricks up their sleeves. We have already seen that in the face of adverse conditions, such as a massive immune response or an attack by antibiotics, the spirochetes quickly change their form to remain undetected. This transformation is an instant, ingrained genetic response and results in the spirochetes changing shape. Spirochetes can either exist in their original worm-like shape or can morph into atypical forms such as round bodies, cystic, rolled, knob-shaped, looped, ring-shaped, globular, and spherical forms. Each of these forms is perfectly able to generate new spirochetes once an attack has passed. Furthermore, in the process of an attack, the spirochetes immediately double the number of round bodies. Scientists believe that this clever transformation takes less than one hour. The longer the attack on them, the more atypical forms the spirochetes develop in response to the adverse environment.

Another one of their nasty tricks is to mess not only with the body but also with the mind of their host. If multiple strains of bacteria have become entrenched and are pervasive in the system, the bacteria can literally take over the mind and consequently the spirit of a person. After having had ample time to study their host, they begin to manipulate the host's hormonal and endocrine system. Once these systems have been hijacked, the bacteria are now able to influence the host in ways that further benefit their survival. They can cause cravings for certain foods, even trigger certain emotions so they can feed off the associated endocrine excretions. At that point, they literally own us.

Despite treatment, encysted forms of the bacteria and spirochete fragments, which contain spirochetal DNA, often remain hidden in the system. And, there is still another way that these clever bacteria can remain undetected––biofilms.

Biofilms are groups of bacteria embedded in gel. Under the motto: *Together we are stronger,* bacteria gather and create a community and then welcome other microbes, including other bacteria, to join them. They know that as a community they have more diversity and can exchange vital information. Therefore, they are better equipped to withstand an attack by antibodies or antibiotics. And––believe it or not––to further remain undetected and so ensure survival, the bacteria continuously alter their structure within the biofilm. Biofilms containing fragments of the spirochetes' DNA embedded in gel have also been found in feces of various infected hosts.

The presence of biofilms as well as spirochete fragments, and remaining encysted spirochetes in the system after treatment, are bad news for the host. They often are found in the brain and central nervous system. Here, they stimulate a continuous immune response, causing ongoing, low-grade infection––chronic Lyme disease.

And then, when you think you have heard it all, there are the blebs––minute granules, almost submicroscopic cellular fractions which have separated from a spirochete's cell. These blebs also contain spirochetal DNA. From the spirochete fragments, biofilms, and blebs, noncultivatable spirochetes eventually emerge. And then––hold onto your seats––if enough time passes, normal, active, cultivatable spirochetes materialize!

Ticks have had a well-oiled relationship with *Borrelia burgdorferi* bacteria. Both the bacteria and the ticks have been around and working together for millions of years. Ticks serve spirochetes by offering a cozy home in their gut, housing up to thirty-five hundred spirochetes per tick. Yuck! Ticks accommodate easy travel for the bacteria with delivery right to the front steps of a variety of hosts, followed by assisted transmission through the ticks' saliva, which is necessary for successful infection.

Spirochetes on the other hand are in many ways responsible for the ticks' thriving. They modify the tick's phenotype—altering its behavior—and so guarantee their own survival. Infected ticks are much more resilient than uninfected ticks. They move quicker, climb higher, are more tolerant to tick repellant, take larger blood meals, store more fat, and stay hydrated longer. They even live longer once infected—up to seven years. And when infected, the Lyme spirochetes supply ticks with a kind of antifreeze, so they can comfortably breeze through the winter. Dang!

Spirochetes are seasoned warriors. They have infected humans for a long time. Lyme spirochetes were detected in an autopsy of Ötzi, the fifty-three hundred-year-old natural mummy found buried in a glacier in the Austrian Alps.

Over the course of their existence, spirochetes have acquired impressive defensive and offensive war strategies. The bacteria have learned how to coordinate information of millions of different processes and use this data to their advantage with precision and reliability, securing the thriving survival of their species. Humbly, we come to realize that our finest technological advances cannot even come close to the spirochetes' intricate, bacterial information-processing capabilities.

Getting rid of ticks will not solve our dilemma either. The *Borrelia burgdorferi* bacteria will simply find a new and probably even more convenient host. These superintelligent pathogens were here long before us and, I suspect, will outlive us with ease.

PART III

TREATMENTS

"Keeping your body healthy is an expression of gratitude
to the whole cosmos;
the trees, the clouds, everything."

—–Thich Nhat Hanh

Treatments for Lyme disease are an ongoing evolving process. With each patient, the disease gives us new symptoms custom tailored by that particular person's immune system and bodily response. Often *Borrelia burgdorferi* is not the only bacterium transmitted through a tick bite. There are other intruders, like *Bartonella*, *Babesia*, *Ehrlichia*, *Powassan virus*, mycoplasmas, *Chlamydia*-like organisms (CLOs), and several more that we know of. New strands are still being discovered. These can be transmitted at the same time as the Lyme bacteria through a bite by arthropods. Some ticks can carry as many as two hundred known infectious microorganisms.

In most hosts, the onslaught of these microorganisms will weaken the immune system. Each host presents a very specific ecosystem to these organisms. And because each body is different, every host responds in a unique way. The response to an infected bite entirely depends on the ability of the immune system to fight the organism. Should the immune system be weakened already, the patient, unable to fight off the intruders, may not only suffer from the effects of Lyme disease but can also become susceptible to a variety of coinfections.

Treating Lyme is not a straightforward process where a certain pharmaceutical or one specific herb is the cure-all. For the practitioner it is rather a process of discovery not unlike the work of a detective. It often involves continual treatment adjustments to a patient's particular symptoms. What works for one person may not work for another person.

TESTING, CONVENTIONAL TREATMENTS, AND ANTIBIOTICS

Antibiotics are the standard treatment in Western medicine for suspected or established Lyme disease. Usually the disease is confirmed by a positive test result or the appearance of a bullseye rash on the patient's skin. Only 30 percent of patients who have been infected by *Borrelia burgdorferi* show a bullseye, as only some of the bacterial genotypes generate it. The bullseye rash is in essence the one absolute proof that Lyme bacteria have indeed infected the host.

To confirm a Lyme disease diagnosis, the most common tests used are the ELISA and the Western blot test. These tests are used in combination; the ELISA test is looking for the *Borrelia burgdorferi* organisms in the blood serum, and the Western blot test is looking for either IgG or IgM antibodies. However, half of all infected people never produce measurable antibodies to Lyme spirochetes, which makes testing for these bacteria difficult. This is the reason why these tests have been shown to be very unreliable, with false negative as well as false positive test results.

There are more reasons than the mere absence of antibodies to make these tests unreliable. The antibodies that are measured by these tests––IgG and IgM antibodies, a specific class of immunoglobulin––refer to proteins that bind to antigens. They are produced by the immune system after an exposure to harmful bacteria. IgM antibodies appear after the third week of infection and are only present for a short amount of time. Afterwards they are often no longer in the bloodstream and therefore will not show up on a test. The IgG antibodies, on the other hand, appear between six weeks and three months after infection. They can linger, even after the patient has recuperated. A test can therefore show a positive Lyme disease result while the person is no longer ill with Lyme disease but instead may suffer from a coinfection. Such a false test result in combination with clinical symptoms can easily lead to misdiagnoses and treatment difficulties.

There is also disagreement among experts on which antibody bands need to be present to indicate a positive test result. Some require as many as five bands to be present to be considered positive for Lyme disease; others look for one or two main bands. In my case, my immune system had produced not merely one or two, nor even five, but a total of ten antibody bands! I guess you could say that I was pretty positive for Lyme disease.

PCR testing, which examines the spirochetal DNA itself, as well as skin biopsies, unfortunately, are also not very effective. Often the number of spirochetes in an afflicted patient appears low because the bacteria are encysted, or inactive at the time, or are well sheltered in hard-to-find niches of the body. In some cases, skin biopsies have produced negative test results even when patients had a visible bullseye rash.

There are also other tests, indicators of variations in blood chemistry, for example. None of them, however, are reliable at this point in time. But a positive Lyme disease test, showing specific Lyme antibodies in conjunction with symptoms a patient exhibits, constitute a good starting point for a clinical Lyme diagnosis.

✳

Doxycycline, a pharmaceutical antibiotic, is typically prescribed if an infection by Lyme bacteria is suspected or confirmed. This antibiotic, which is taken orally, is considered to be the most successful pharmaceutical drug for all Lyme-related diseases at the time of this writing. Depending on the number of days that have passed since the tick bite and occurrence of infection, either a ten-day, two-week, or a four-week round of Doxycycline is the norm.

Understanding the bacterium as well as the coinfectious pathogens explains why results of treatments with antibiotics are inconsistent. Antibiotics attach themselves to bacterial cell walls in order to kill the bacterium. In the face of adversity, *Borrelia burgdorferi* bacteria have the ability to collapse their cell walls around themselves, creating a cloaking device. Transformed, the bacteria are no longer detectable by antibiotics, the body's own immune system, or by tests.

Confronted with unpleasant conditions caused by the presence of antibiotics in the bloodstream, the bacteria further attempt to escape from the threat and seek cover in hard-to-find places. By using their worm-like behavior, they bury themselves deeply into tissue where blood flow is scarce. Hidden from their attackers, they proceed to change their form further and then hibernate. During their time of hibernation, they have a much-reduced metabolism—they do not feed or reproduce. The bacteria are in fact in an altered morphological state. For the host, symptoms appear to have disappeared. In reality, the bacteria are not idle at all while hibernating. They are busy learning the host's unique immune system and the characteristics of their attackers. They are in fact molding themselves—changing their DNA—to become more resilient until it is time to reemerge.

The sophisticated defense strategy of the bacteria, the ability to transform into round bodies, encysted forms, or biofilms—the hardest-to-kill bacterial form—turns the bacterial cells into so-called "persister" cells, rendering them tolerant toward antibiotics. It assures the bacteria a high survival rate. These microorganisms have been termed "masters of illusiveness" for good reason. They can remain in hibernation in encysted form for up to three years, or until the environment is free of pressure from attackers and it is safe for the bacteria to reemerge.

Long-term antibiotic treatments may keep the organisms at a low level in the body, falsely giving the impression that the infection has subsided. In most cases antibiotic treatments are unable to eradicate the bacteria completely. It is not uncommon, when long-term antibiotic treatments are finally discontinued, for spirochetes to reemerge from hibernation and to become active again.

Thus, Doxycycline has been shown to be a powerful attacker, but also has considerable downsides. Another problem with antibiotics is their inability to reach the bacteria once it has left the bloodstream. Antibiotics are generally unable to travel to those places in the body where bacteria like to hang out. Only in extremely high doses, or when infusions of antibiotics are administered intravenously, can the medication reach the brain or spinal cord. Still, studies have shown a relapse rate of nearly 35 percent of patients treated "successfully" with antibiotics.

When choosing antibiotics as treatment for Lyme disease, it is important to consider the potential damage that high amounts of antibiotics can do to the body itself. Antibiotics kill bacteria, good and bad, and so disrupt gut health and digestion, and consequently weaken the immune system. The use of antibiotics further encourages a natural, genetic evolution toward resistance within the bacteria: as we have seen, *Borrelia burgdorferi* is highly adaptive. In this sense, antibiotics have a mixed effect on Lyme disease. On the one hand, they are capable of killing 90 percent of the spirochetes during an early infection-- yet on the other hand, their presence in the bloodstream causes spirochetes to double the number of round bodies that are being produced and prompts the bacteria to develop resistance. Unfortunately for us, it is highly possible that *Borrelia burgdorferi* will eventually become resilient to Doxycycline and other types of antibiotics.

There are studies in the works today to combine either two antibiotics, or an antibiotic and another chemical (such as an antihistaminic drug), to inhibit the bacteria's ability to evolve and change form over time to ensure that the round bodies are structurally deformed or killed. Hopefully, useful results will emerge soon. Considering what information is available today, we know that antibiotics can significantly reduce the symptoms of Lyme disease but cannot completely kill off all the bacteria in most cases.

Duration of infection is crucial. The longer the bacteria have been in the body, the greater the chance that they will not respond to antibiotics or other drugs and become harder to eradicate. While untreated, the bacteria have a chance to learn and adjust to the specific immune system of the host, which gives them the know-how to reproduce in a way that makes their offspring more resilient and capable of survival. A wrong dose of pharmaceuticals and other drugs, or too short a dosing period can have the same effect.

Despite the fact that a core group of 25 to 40 percent of infected people do not respond to antibiotics or relapse after treatment, it is important to mention that, in other cases, especially where the infection is detected within hours or days from bacterial transmission, *antibiotics can be very effective*. Many people can be cured by the use of antibiotics if administered immediately upon infection while the bacteria are still in the bloodstream.

HERBAL TREATMENTS

"The natural healing force within us
is the greatest force in getting well."

—Hippocrates

Before I dive into available herbal treatments for Lyme disease, let me introduce you to two experts in the field who have contributed tremendously to my understanding of Lyme disease and how to treat it with the healing power of plants.

STEPHEN HARROD BUHNER

I discovered Stephen Harrod Buhner when desperately searching for alternative methods to heal myself from Lyme disease after a failure with antibiotics. Buhner has studied Lyme disease for over thirty-five years. He has written several books on healing Lyme and many other books on related topics. Buhner has had contact with over twenty-five thousand people infected with Lyme bacteria within the last decade alone and has had extensive in-depth treatment experiences with hundreds of patients during that time. His meticulous research on Lyme disease, coinfections, treatments, and outcomes includes reviews of nearly ten thousand peer-reviewed journal papers. I consider Buhner an absolute authority on healing Lyme and a genius when it comes to understanding the healing power of plants.

I have studied Buhner's book *Healing Lyme* as if it were my Lyme disease bible. I inhaled its information and applied its recommendations. Sprinkled with Latin terms and medical journal excerpts, this is not a casual read. However, I highly recommend *Healing Lyme* to anyone who wants to know everything about Lyme *Borreliosis* and its coinfections. I especially recommend *Healing Lyme* as a reference manual for clinicians.

TIMOTHY LEE SCOTT

It is no surprise that in my research about Lyme disease I eventually came across Timothy Lee Scott. Tim is the author of *Invasive Plant Medicine*, and is a former student of Stephen Harrod Buhner. He is a health care practitioner with a background in Chinese medicine, acupuncture, and herbalism. He is also a writer and researcher.

Tim has been treating patients afflicted with Lyme disease since 2004. I have had the pleasure to meet him personally and learn about his experience with Lyme disease.

Tim's Story

As an avid outdoorsman and herbalist, Tim loves to spend time in nature. Pulling off a creepy crawly after a day outside is nothing unusual.

One summer, when he caught the flu, he did not think much about it. However unfortunate, it would be better after the typical seven days of aching and fighting a fever. But after a couple of days of flu-like symptoms, Tim experienced unusual and intense neck pain. And instead of getting better over the course of the following week, he awoke one morning feeling as if he had aged fifty years overnight. At that point he realized that he had more than the flu. The reason for the painful symptoms, he concluded, must have been a tick he had pulled off a couple of weeks earlier. He knew he had been hit hard with Lyme disease.

Immediately, he put himself on herbal remedies, as, after all, herbs are his specialty. And as he expected, he regained his health quickly. Three months after the onset of Lyme disease he was feeling great and believed himself to be fully recuperated. Unaware at the time of the devious nature of the *Borrelia burgdorferi* bacteria, he stopped taking the herbs.

But soon after, he relapsed––not uncommon for Lyme disease patients. This time he got severely ill, however, much worse than the first time. He suffered from headaches, fatigue, and achy joints, interwoven with emotional ups and downs. Symptoms so severe that Tim was unable to work. Still the disease progressed, and eventually he was laid up in bed.

Tim continued the herbal protocol under forced rest. These were hard times. It took another six months until he began seeing glimpses of his old self, was able to move a little, even dared a short walk around the house. Yet he still was not able to exert himself without suffering repercussions. Just walking up his driveway became a major goal. If he pushed himself too hard, he would pay for it dearly the next day. Finally, as his body began to heal, he had a little more energy and experienced fewer symptoms. It took a total of thirteen months until he recuperated from this relapse.

But the world of ticks, bacteria, and Lyme disease is an unscrupulous world. Tim was back one hundred percent and doing great when he was bitten again. This time he did not wait for symptoms. Instead, he chose a proactive route and responded quickly and aggressively with the herbal protocol. He took strong and extended doses. Still, he suffered from strange symptoms, different from what he had experienced before. These were symptoms atypical for Lyme, but, as he soon discovered, symptoms typical for coinfections common to Lyme disease. Ticks carry up to two hundred strains of bacteria which often make it hard to impossible to diagnose the actual disease. Realizing, however, that he suffered from a coinfection, Tim adjusted his herbal protocol and subsequently got better.

There was something puzzling about this situation, however, something that did not quite make sense to Tim. Tim had spent ample time outside in fields and woods on a regular basis. Being bitten by a tick was nothing unusual. And, in all likelihood, some of these previous ticks which had latched on to him had also been infected with *Borrelia burgdorferi* or other strains of harmful bacteria. What was different with this tick bite compared to previous bites?

Pondering this question, Tim realized that, during the time he contracted Lyme disease, he had actually made himself susceptible to disease. He had been working as a practitioner and raising a one-year-old, while also building a house and supporting a family. Naturally, he had been stressed and run-down in the face of such a heavy load. In hindsight, it was easy to see that he had had too much on his plate. Whereas a healthy immune system can fight even *Borrelia burgdorferi* successfully without pharmaceuticals or herbs, a stressed and weakened immune system is unable to do so.

Stress is detrimental to our health. It sneaks its way slowly into our lives, mostly undetected until it has established itself. We usually don't go from a well-balanced life to a stressed-out life overnight. Just like the frog that does not realize the water is getting too hot to sit in while the temperature slowly rises, we often don't recognize that stress is making its way into our lives until we experience repercussions.

In our go-go world, where the emphasis is on doing, to rest and to do nothing is frowned upon. We feel guilty even just thinking of doing nothing for a short while. Meanwhile, studies show that sleep and rest are essential building blocks necessary for a healthy body and mind. Resting allows the body to recharge itself on a cellular level. We understand that rest and sleep are essential to any healing process, but they are also prerequisites to remaining healthy. Rest keeps the immune system strong and able to do its job. While in our fast-moving society we look down upon rest, it is as important to our wellbeing as oxygen.

As my uncle Emil once said, if you are stressed and have no time, take one hour to rest. And if you are experiencing a day where you absolutely have no time at all, then take two!

His illness forced Tim to find a balance between rest, daily life, and exercise. Like most of us who live in a busy world, Tim was unaware before being struck with Lyme disease how stressed he was and what resting truly meant. It was normal for him to work all day and then, once home, continue to work in the garden or elsewhere around the house. Maybe after dinner he would allow himself to watch a movie. Like most of us, that was also his idea of resting. Not until he was flat on his back did he come to understand the meaning and importance of rest.

Laid up in bed, Tim had much time to contemplate. Rest was no longer a choice. Resting allows our mind to become quiet. Once the usual jabbering in the head subsides, we actually awaken and become alert to a deeper truth, the microscopic things that reside deep within us. While resting, Tim not only began to heal, but also to notice these subtle gifts within and all around for which we normally have little time.

As Tim gradually began to recuperate, he learned that rest needed to remain a part of his life. Exerting himself created only issues and setbacks, and consequently slowed down recovery and jeopardized his health. The illness had become a teacher for Tim.

Tim also kept a journal during his recovery, which turned out to be very helpful. When struck with Lyme, it can become difficult to remember what happened earlier in the day, let alone a few days ago. Keeping a journal can show that we are indeed making progress, even though we may not feel it at the time. When still struggling after six months, Tim went back and read his prior entries. He realized that he was at least not as bad as he had been. In fact, he was much better than during the onset of the disease. This gave hope, encouragement, and confidence in his treatment.

✳

Since his recovery, and to no one's surprise, Tim has been bitten a few more times by a tick. But with an immediate and targeted response, he has had no reoccurrences or any symptoms of Lyme disease.

Having suffered from Lyme disease, Tim can truly relate to the agony that patients who are struck by the disease endure. Helping others to recuperate from Lyme disease has become Tim's focus in his practice. Today, Tim is a practitioner who specializes in treating Lyme and other chronic diseases.

As an herbalist, he has a deep understanding of the ecological benefits as well as the healing abilities of medicinal plants, including invasives. His love for the healing power of these plants, as well as the growing need for herbal remedies, has prompted him to create Green Dragon Botanicals (www.GreenDragonBotanicals.com) in Vermont, where he can be reached.

MEDICINAL PLANTS

"Extreme remedies are very appropriate
for extreme diseases."

—Hippocrates

The herbal remedies addressed (including dosages) in this chapter are a combination of Buhner's and Scott's recommendations, both of which formed the basis of my recovery. Of course, there are most certainly many more medicinal plants with potential healing power for Lyme disease than are mentioned here. The herbal remedies discussed below are only those which I have used with great success. The full protocol and exact dosages I took are listed in the Appendix. These dosages worked for me; however, with herbal supplements, often dosages suggest a range rather than an exact amount. If the immune system is healthy, a smaller amount will probably suffice. For a depleted immune system, a larger amount may be needed. If severely affected by the disease and sensitive to these substances, a tiny amount should be tested and then slowly increased over time. If embarking on this journey without the guidance of a practitioner, it is important to listen to one's intuition.

Healing Plants and Why We Need Them

Over the millions of years that plants have been around, bacteria have been around as well. During their coexistence, bacteria and plants have had a mutual exchange of information. Plants have learned how to deal with bacteria and their various forms, including biofilms. Plants understand how to tune into their environment, read temperature and climate, distinguish between characteristics of their bacterial attackers as well as benefactors, and change their plant chemistry accordingly. Being able to understand what is happening in their environment, plants are able to respond in a self-preserving way and communicate this information not only to each other but also to other plant life and possibly to certain microorganisms. They know how to fine-tune their defense mechanisms. Recent research has confirmed that plants indeed do communicate with one another.

There is more going on than just a local response to environmental conditions among plants. There is an intelligence at play that encourages plant migration. Plants migrate not only because of weather and temperature changes but also for other, more subtle reasons.

It has been observed that the invasive plant Japanese knotweed, a plant that is highly effective in treating Lyme disease, moves into an area, or, if already present, begins to spread rapidly about five to ten years prior to the appearance of Lyme disease. Where Japanese knotweed has become invasive in the United States happens to be the same states where Lyme disease has moved in.

Japanese knotweed is a powerful healing plant for us, but also for the environment. It loves to grow along roadsides, former waste sites, and along wastewater runoffs. It has the ability to absorb zinc, lead, and copper in its plant body. It is a virtual vacuum cleaner for pollutants.

Plants' Databank of Information

Plants' enormous databank of information on how to navigate their way around bacteria can be a powerful tool and is the reason for our using them as a healing modality. Understanding their power, we use plants for various purposes. Medicinal plants can function on their own as a healing herb, or they can function as a support for the healing properties of other herbs. They can also assist the function of pharmaceuticals––literally intensifying the effects of an antibiotic.

Whereas an antibiotic works with a single chemical compound, or possibly two or three compounds, herbs have multiple chemistries at play. Because of their immense experience with bacteria, they have hundreds of different compounds which work synergistically together to address an infection. Herbs can be anti-inflammatory, antibacterial, antiviral, antifungal, antispirochetal, antioxidant, antiulcer, and so many more properties all in one! They work with a person's immune system with an array of compounds and fight an infection holistically. They support the body's own immune system and aid in the detoxification process at the same time.

Plants have stored the information on how to address disease in the databank of their DNA. For this reason, plants have been used by humankind for thousands of years through various cultures and have left us with quite a bit of history to work with. Plants have millions of years of experience, and they are good at what they are doing. We are lucky to have them available to support our wellbeing.

Bacteria have not been idle either, over the course of history. They have absorbed the changes of the environment and the changes in their food sources, continually adding information to their extensive resource library. They have learned how to circumvent the defense mechanisms of plants and, later, animals, and finally humans. The challenge for us is to understand which herb has what quality and healing potential to fight off the bacteria. Luckily, much of this wisdom has been passed down through generations, first orally and then in writing, and is available to us today.

I am grateful to incredible and dedicated people like Stephen Harrod Buhner, Timothy Lee Scott, and so many others who have researched and studied the knowledge of plants and their healing powers, and have then gone about organizing the information in a way that lay people can understand and make good use of it. Without their meticulous work, this valuable knowledge could one day be lost.

The Immune System and Borrelia burgdorferi

It all begins with saliva. Once a tick bites and a trace of saliva enters the blood stream of a host, a devious process begins. The saliva's immune-inhibiting molecules cause the imminent immune response by the host to become dormant. This is a convenient way for the spirochetes to undertake a stealth attack, the first of many highly sophisticated tricks.

Without an immune response, the bacteria have free range to infect and cultivate their new host. They begin by circulating in the bloodstream and lymphatic system, where they float to the nearest lymph nodes. They aim for the spleen, liver, heart, and bone marrow. While busy altering the immune response in the lymph nodes, they can continue their journey to the brain and central nervous system where often the most severe damage is done.

The host's immune system is not ignorant when it comes to responding to such an attack. Humans have been around for hundreds of thousands of years, maybe even longer, and have learned over time how to respond to bacterial attacks. Atypical forms of bacteria––encysted forms, round bodies, and biofilms––have also been around for a very long time. Our immune system knows how to deal with these forms of bacteria, provided that the immune system is healthy. It knows how to get rid of them. The immune system is not a static system, either. It continuously learns and adds information to its databank. After having successfully fought off a bacterial intruder, it is unlikely that another attack by the *same* bacterial strain will lead to infection. Other strains, of course, may still succeed.

People with healthy immune systems can be infected by Lyme spirochetes yet show only a few symptoms––or no symptoms at all. A healthy body will clear the infection very quickly. If our immune system is compromised, however, we will likely fall victim to a bacterial attack and possibly suffer from an infection and, unfortunately, often long-lasting, debilitating consequences.

Buhner gives us hope and good news by letting us know that a healthy immune system is not only able to kill off the intruder, but will immediately produce corresponding antibodies. These antibodies, produced in response to the presence of a specific bacteria in the blood stream, will cause future ticks to dislike this host and drop before they will feed, forcing them to begin a new search for a more palatable meal. A high number of antibody bands indicates that the immune system is healthy and working full tilt, having sent out its army to kill off the invaders.

The ten antibody bands found in my blood serum during testing should have been an indication to health care providers that my immune system was winning the battle with Lyme bacteria, especially considering the fact that I was feeling great at the time, showing no symptoms whatsoever of any illness. Instead, I was diagnosed with a case of *severe* Lyme disease and put on an extended round of Doxycycline, which destroyed all that my immune system had accomplished.

The problem is that most of us do not have a healthy and strong immune system at all times. Stress alone can weaken it enough to render it unable to respond appropriately to a stealth attack by a vicious bacterium such as *Borrelia burgdorferi*. The weaker the immune system, the easier it is for microbes to infest and infect a host, and the more severe the symptoms will be.

In essence, a healthy and strong immune system can fight off intruding attackers such as the Lyme spirochetes without pharmaceutical or herbal assistance. It is then our first priority to keep our immune system healthy. If it is weakened, our goal must be to strengthen it and nurture it back to optimal health. The second priority is to assist the body in dealing with the debilitating symptoms of Lyme disease and to restore where damage has already occurred.

Specific Medicinal Plants - The Next Line of Defense

The healing power of plants may well be the most powerful weapon we have when it comes to eliminating *Borrelia burgdorferi* bacteria. We can use these plants in a very specific way. The first contact we have with spirochetes is through the saliva of the tick. As we have already learned, tick saliva inactivates and inhibits the immune response, which allows spirochetes to infect our body undetected. Luckily, we know of plants that have the ability to protect us from these intruders and effectively shut the gates on them. As previously mentioned, it is best to proceed under the guidance of a skilled practitioner to choose the correct combination of herbs and the right dosage. Herbs are very powerful healers but improperly used can also cause severe side effects.

Astragalus

Astragalus is an immune-potentiating herb, which greatly counteracts those factors introduced by tick saliva, inhibiting an immune response. By specifically supporting the part of the immune response that is inactivated or inhibited by tick saliva, the risk of an infection by spirochetes can be significantly reduced.

Buhner suggests taking this herb on a regular basis as part of the diet if living in an endemic region (1000 mg daily), or to add it to the diet during tick-feeding cycles (3000 mg daily). (More about ticks and their feeding cycles can be found in Part II of this book, "Ticks and *Borrelia Burgdorferi*.")

Buhner mentions in his revised edition of *Healing Lyme* that in some cases Astragalus can worsen the condition during *chronic* Lyme. If symptoms worsen once Astragalus is added to the protocol, it should be discontinued.

Japanese Knotweed

When spirochetes first enter the blood and the lymph channels, they are being transported via the bloodstream and lymphatic system to various organs. Once they have reached their preferred cells or tissue compartments in the host, the spirochetes use adhesions to target molecules. Their favorite molecules are cartilage and collagen, which are present throughout the body. Always hungry, the bacteria then release a substance (their poop--yech!) which breaks down these molecules. Once broken down, they become nutrients for the spirochetes.

With cartilage and collagen damaged, our bodily structure becomes weakened. Without any additional stress put on the body, Lyme disease patients often suffer from unexplainable, sudden ruptures of tendons and ligaments, or throw out their back.

Unfortunately, I am only too familiar with this scenario. After a failed treatment with antibiotics, spirochetes that had managed to successfully hide out in hidden corners of my body made a comeback. During that time, I suddenly became super flexible. It felt as though my joints were loose. I was able to bend my body in ways I had not managed in decades despite regular stretching and yoga. And then my back went out. Spirochetes had successfully broken down cartilage and collagen in my body, to a point where it could no longer hold itself together.

Spirochetes also aim to break down tissue by creating inflammation. They have a sophisticated way to accomplish this. When bacteria touch certain proteins in the brain, the immune system instantly responds and produces inflammatory cytokines--nonantibody proteins. The job of these cytokines is to kill off the bacteria. Meanwhile, the bacteria release their own cytokines to cause inflammation and tissue breakdown. During long-term brain infection, *Borrelia burgdorferi* continually stimulate proteins in the brain, encouraging the release of inflammatory cytokines. Under this constant threat, the immune system becomes overactive, fighting back with a cytokine cascade and increasing inflammation evermore. The bacteria are using our own immune response to their advantage. On the one hand, they cleverly decrease parts of the immune system function in order to go about their business undetected, causing inflammation along the way. On the other hand, the bacteria purposely activate an immune response, knowing that this will further increase inflammation. They accomplish exactly what they want—creating more and more inflammation and so securing an ample food supply for themselves.

Buhner tells us that Japanese knotweed is the herb of choice to interrupt this process. The weed has the ability to block the proteins' expression of inflammatory cytokines and to inhibit every one of the spirochetes' upregulated cytokines. Japanese knotweed protects the brain structures from inflammatory damage. As an inhibitor, it counteracts the process of tissue breakdown and so prevents the advance of the bacteria further into the body.

Japanese knotweed further has the capability to cross the gastrointestinal tract barrier and the blood-brain barrier. This is significant, as spirochetes cross the blood-brain barrier to move to various hard-to-find places in the body, especially the central nervous system and the brain. Having taken up residence in the central nervous system, the bacteria then proceed to break down the myelin sheaths that surround the nerves. Spirochetes prefer to attach themselves to specific parts of these protective myelin sheaths. They like the places where there is a natural gap in the sheaths. This location—a pathway—is a favorite spot for spirochetes to gain nutrients.

During the process of creating a meal for themselves by breaking down the myelin sheaths, components of these myelin sheaths begin to float into spaces in the brain where they do not belong. Alarmed, the immune system responds by attacking these fragments. With the ongoing presence of these components in the brain, however, the immune system gets overwhelmed and begins to register all myelin sheaths as foreign bodies. As a result, it ends up attacking not just the floating components but healthy myelin sheaths as well.

The overactive immune response in conglomeration with the spirochete-generated cytokines as well as the immune-response-generated cytokines can result in massive damage to the brain. The continuous loss of myelin sheaths causes many symptoms found in autoimmune conditions. This is the reason why Lyme disease patients are often misdiagnosed with autoimmune disorders.

The neuro-structures of the brain can be protected, however, if levels of inflammatory cytokines can be reduced and the breakdown of myelin sheaths prevented. Japanese knotweed has the ability to reduce the number of spirochete-induced cytokines, as well as to inhibit easy access to the pathways the bacteria prefer.

Japanese knotweed acts as a powerful antimicrobial and anti-inflammatory agent. It has the capability of reaching difficult areas and hard-to-find niches in the body. It protects the brain from bacterial infection and microbial damage and inhibits the pathways spirochetes use in order to gain nutrition. It is the number one plant Buhner recommends for stopping damage caused by *Borrelia burgdorferi*, particularly in the nervous system.

Among its other components, Japanese knotweed contains high amounts of resveratrol. It actually contains the most resveratrol of any plant known, including the famous pinot noir grape ––a good excuse to have a glass of red wine now and then. Resveratrol is known to be beneficial for the heart, joints, brain, skin, and is very good at reducing inflammation in general. Many life-enhancing claims are attributed to resveratrol.

If using resveratrol tablets to treat Lyme disease, it is important to make sure it comes from the Japanese knotweed root and not from the grape, as resveratrol alone is not enough to treat Lyme disease. Buhner says that all plant components of Japanese Knotweed––which work in synergy––are necessary to successfully treat the disease.

Japanese knotweed has many more benefits. It spreads easily throughout the body and reaches areas such as the eye, heart, skin, and joints––places where blood flow is limited and spirochetes prefer to take residence. Just as Japanese knotweed itself seems to migrate to geographic areas where Lyme disease is spreading, in our body, its healing components seem to seek those places where Lyme bacteria have settled.

Japanese knotweed also enhances the movement of herbal compounds throughout the body, acting as an herb synergist. When taken together with other herbs and/ or pharmaceutical drugs, it facilitates the movement of these substances into the far-to-reach places of the body. It contains high amounts of vitamin C and functions as a powerful antioxidant.

Japanese knotweed truly is the queen of all medicinal plants when it comes to healing Lyme disease. More complete information can be found in Buhner's *Healing Lyme* as well as in the Appendix. Recommended dosage: ¼ tsp. to 1 tsp. in the form of a tincture, 3 to 6 times daily.

CAT'S CLAW, GINKGO BILOBA, AND LION'S MANE

When spirochetes enter the central nervous system and brain, they modulate the production and release of cytokines and other chemical molecules. These potent substances cause inflammation, increase the effect and power of free radicals, and eventually cause the death of neurons.

Once the neural system has been damaged, it is a slow process to restore health. However, the good news is that neural restoration is possible, especially in younger patients. Buhner assures us that neural damage caused by *Borrelia burgdorferi* is reversible! The regeneration of these structures is a process that will take time, however—six months to three years. One has to be patient.

There are many herbs that can assist in protecting the neural structures and reversing neural damage. Cat's claw is one of the most potent herbs used to protect the brain from the effects of these toxic substances as well as to reduce their levels in the brain.

Cat's claw is also an immune system supporter and is a helpful herb in the treatment of arthritic conditions and joint health. Recommended dosage: ¼ to ½ tsp. in the form of a tincture, 3 times daily.

Chinese cat's claw, a slightly different variety from regular cat's claw, is specific to neurological issues caused by Lyme disease. It easily crosses the blood brain barrier and it is also often used for headaches, eye issues, and Bell's palsy. Recommended dosage: ½ tsp. to 1 tsp. in the form of a tincture, 3 to 6 times daily.

Ginkgo biloba is useful for decreased blood flow to the brain. Recommended dosage: 1 tsp in the form of a tincture., 3 to 6 times daily. (Caution: this herb could cause excess bleeding.)

And to stimulate neural *re*growth, the mushroom Lion's Mane has proven to be helpful. Since news about the health benefits of Lion's Mane has become known, a movement of underground mushroom growers has begun to sprout in basements all over the nation.

Hyaluronic Acid

Hyaluronic acid is found throughout our bodily tissues. Spirochetes like to attach themselves to and degrade hyaluronic acid. This degradation allows spirochetes to penetrate further into the body. The breakdown of hyaluronic acid is the cause of many Lyme disease symptoms.

Including hyaluronic acid in a treatment protocol can be tremendously helpful. It adds back what the spirochetes haven taken out. Skin repairs itself by using hyaluronic acid. Buhner assures that collagen damaged by *Borrelia* spirochetes can heal and regrow better and faster the more hyaluronic acid is present. Recommended dosage: 1 Tablespoon daily in the form of a tincture.

Echinacea Angustifolia

The process of creating the substance the *Borrelia burgdorferi* bacteria release to soften and break down connective tissue can be slowed and stopped by the use of an inhibitor.

If the bodily tissues and the structure of mucus and skin membranes remain strong, bacteria are unable to move further into the body. Echinacea works as an inhibitor and is helpful in preventing the breakdown of bodily tissues. Recommended dosage: 1 tsp. in the form of a tincture, 3 to 6 times daily.

ANDROGRAPHIS, JAPANESE KNOTWEED, RED SAGE, AND CHINESE SKULLCAP

A small portion of *Borrelia burgdorferi* bacteria immediately form biofilms upon entering the host. This ensures a high rate of survival for the bacteria. Biofilms are difficult to eradicate and are antibiotic tolerant. They are the underlying cause for the long-term, chronic conditions of Lyme disease. Some biofilms are healthy biofilms, however, and it is important not to destroy these in our gut while attempting to eradicate the unwanted ones.

Plants have been dealing with bacterial biofilms for millions of years. They have learned how to successfully get rid of them and have stored this know-how in their DNA. Over time, and with an adequate dose, herbs can break down unwanted biofilms until they are completely eradicated.

Andrographis, Japanese Knotweed, and Chinese Skullcap are powerful agents that have the capability to break down biofilms. If used over time, these herbs will reduce the number of bacteria in biofilms and ultimately inhibit the formation of new biofilms. They do so gently, until the unwanted biofilms are completely removed from the body. Buhner recommends combining Japanese Knotweed with Red Sage and Chinese Skullcap for best results: Recommended dosage: Japanese Knotweed, ¼ to 1 tsp. in the form of a tincture, 3 to 6 times daily. Red Sage and Chinese Skullcap, 1 tsp. each in the form of a tincture, 3 times a day.

In order for an herb to be an effective agent against spirochetes, it has to be extremely systemic--working throughout the entire body--and it has to be antibacterial for every single variety of bacterial form that the *Borrelia burgdorferi* spirochete generates of itself. Andrographis is a powerful, broad-spectrum herbal antibiotic and antibacterial agent. It is very active against intracellular bacteria, reduces cytokines, and breaks up biofilms. It has the ability to cross the blood-brain barrier and to reach the bacteria hiding out in the farthest corners of the body.

Andrographis can be very effective as an antibacterial for about sixty percent of patients. However, in some rare situations––in about one percent of cases where Andrographis has been used––the herb has caused severe hives. This herb should be taken with caution and only under the supervision of a skilled practitioner. Recommended dosage: 600 mg, 3 times a day for one week. If no side effects, increase to 1,200 mg, 3 times a day.

Andrographis––as a bacteria killer––is also a great and effective remedy to use externally. In the form of a tincture, it can be put directly on a tick bite once the tick is removed to reduce the number of bacteria attempting to enter the body.

Teasel

Teasel is a plant that has been used in herbal medicine around the world for centuries. From old literature we learn that teasel's qualities lend themselves to the treatment of gout, arthritis, rheumatism, hepatitis, and gallbladder ailments. Teasel tastes bitter, reminding us of stomach bitters. It has flushing, detoxifying, and anti-inflammatory qualities that greatly assist the kidneys and the liver. It is often used to help with digestion.

Recently, especially in Europe, teasel has become the herbal remedy of choice for treating Lyme disease. Often, teasel root is the only remedy prescribed when treating Lyme disease with an herbal treatment protocol.

Teasel is a prickly thistle. When flowering, it creates a ring of blossoms around its flower head. This ring eventually splits into two rings, where one moves toward the top of the egg-shaped flower head and the other moves toward the bottom. Interestingly, the movements of these rings in the flowering teasel remind us of the so-called bullseye rash—the typical sign of a Borrelial infection—which sometimes appears around a tick bite and ever so slowly expands outward.

The qualities of the teasel plant can be absorbed through various methods. When making tea, the roots and the leaves are steamed. This is ideal when working with children. Teasel tincture is made from fresh teasel root and usually made with alcohol. Root powder is another way to acquire the healing properties of this plant. The powder is bitter and best mixed with honey.

Interestingly, teasel has been shown to work well as treatment for Lyme disease in Europe and in the Midwest of the United States. In both these areas, teasel grows abundantly. It does not seem to be as effective as a treatment in the Northeast of the United States, where it hardly grows.

I was infected by Lyme disease in the Northeast of the United States. Later, after my unsuccessful treatment with antibiotics, I visited my family in Europe, where I learned about teasel. Immediately, I began my first herbal treatment with a homeopathic remedy of teasel extract. This worked well but did not seem to be able to cure me completely. Later, after much research, I concluded that the reason teasel was unable to completely heal my infection, was probably because I had been infected with Lyme spirochetes in the Northeast of the United States. Ticks can carry up to two hundred different strains of bacteria. Some of these strains may well be unique to ticks in specific areas. It may be possible that the strains in Europe and in the Midwest of the United States differ from the strains that ticks carry in the Northeast. Medicinal plants seem to grow mysteriously where they are most effective. Teasel does hardly grow in the Northeast and does not seem to be as effective in healing Lyme disease in that region compared to areas where it is native and abundant.

Recommended dosage: 20 to 30 drops, 3 times a day as a tincture; or 5 drops, 3 times a day in form of a homeopathic remedy.

Final Thoughts on Herbal Treatments

When the body is infiltrated with destructive organisms such as spirochetes, it is important to address the situation in multiple ways. Parts of the herbal treatment are aimed at lessening the symptoms of the disease, blocking the bacteria from migrating deeper into the body or changing form. Other parts of the treatment need to be aimed at supporting and strengthening the immune system and the body's adrenal response. A well-rounded herbal protocol addresses all areas. If all bases are covered, the bacteria experience continuous pressure and eventually are unable to feed or multiply.

An herbal protocol can typically span a time period of eight to twelve months or even longer. It is not a quick fix, but rather a slow and steady rebuilding of the immune system and healing of the damage done by the bacteria. Timothy Scott recommends a re-evaluation three months into treatment. If the situation has not improved by then, potential coinfections or other underlying illnesses need to be considered and the treatment protocol adjusted accordingly.

Spirochetes have the ability to remain in hibernation for up to three years. They linger in the hard-to-find places of the body, encapsulated, undetectable, and cleverly adjusting their DNA to the host's immune-defense capabilities. If pressure is kept on them by medicinal plants, the bacteria have to continue to wait. However, after a maximum time of three years, they need to feed or they will die off. It is therefore advisable to stay on a core regimen of preventative herbs for up to three years from the beginning of treatment, in case some spirochetes are still present in the body.

During tick season, and if living in an area that is infested with ticks, it is a good idea to take preventative, immune-strengthening herbs as a first line of defense. Japanese knotweed and astragalus lend themselves to this task very well, as they are excellent immune-supportive herbs.

Herbs are usually well tolerated. However, some herbs, or too much of an herb, may cause unpleasant reactions in some people. It is recommended to start out with a low dose of medicinal herbs and gradually increase the dose over time. The goal is to find the body's maximum tolerance for the herb and so enjoy maximum healing benefits. The exact dose often varies from person to person. The precise quantity of a particular dose in most herbs is probably not as important as the actual information that is contained in the DNA of the plant.

Digestive upsets are the biggest indicator that one has reached and exceeded the maximum tolerance. It is a sign to back off and reduce the dose to where the body was last able to tolerate the herbs.

HYPERBARIC OXYGEN THERAPY

"The first wealth is health."

--Ralph Waldo Emerson

I was introduced to the healing capabilities of the hyperbaric oxygen chamber by Dr. Grace Johnstone. While sitting in Grace's sunroom, nestled into the corner of a comfortable couch and listening to her story, it was hard for me to imagine that this woman--so radiant and full of energy-- had been terribly sick not too long ago.

GRACE'S STORY

A few years before I met Grace, she was hosting a dinner at her house when she suddenly felt strange. Something was off. She felt feverish but tried to stay focused on being a good host until the evening came to a close. Exhausted, she fell into bed hoping that she would wake up feeling better the next morning.

The following day, Grace awoke feeling extremely ill. Her fever was much higher and she suffered from intense head pain. She suspected that she had caught a virus. A trip to the ER confirmed her suspicion––meningitis.

It was expected that Grace would recover significantly within a week. But she did not get better during the days that followed her visit to the emergency room. Instead, the symptoms worsened dramatically, demanding another trip to the ER. She was prescribed morphine to ease the pain, and an appointment was scheduled with her primary caregiver.

During that appointment Grace noticed that she had developed rashes on her body. It had been about ten days since the onset of the illness. Suspicious, her primary caregiver sent images of the rashes to an expert at the center of infectious diseases at a major hospital. From the images and Grace's symptoms, the expert concluded that Grace was suffering from Lyme meningitis.

Meningitis is an inflammation of the membranes that outline the brain and spinal cord. *Viral* meningitis is caused by viruses common during summer and fall. The viruses, once contracted, begin to multiply in the digestive tract and then spread through the body causing meningitis. *Bacterial* meningitis is a more severe form of the infection and can cause serious damage to the brain, sometimes even death. Lyme meningitis is one of the bacterial infections. It is caused by the Lyme bacterium, is extremely painful, but usually not fatal.

At the time of the diagnosis, Grace had endured a persistent fever of 104°F and was no longer able to stay hydrated. She was admitted to the hospital and prescribed intravenous antibiotics for a duration of two weeks––the standard protocol for Lyme meningitis. After two weeks, Grace was better than she had been, yet clearly not well. The doctors extended the protocol to a full month of IV antibiotics. When the treatment was finished, Grace was able to return home.

Grace had been severely weakened by the illness and month-long stay in the hospital. Once home, she focused on restoring her depleted body. Yet before long, she began to suffer from intense back pain for no apparent reason. The back pain was followed by abdominal pain, then pain in her leg so strong that Grace was no longer able to use her flexor muscles. The restriction allowed her to walk only sideways. Several more trips to the ER resulted in no logical diagnosis. Doctors tested for other conditions––a ruptured ovary, ulcerating fibroids. They were sure it could not be Lyme since Grace had already received a full month of IV antibiotics which was believed to have killed all Lyme bacteria for certain.

Unable to present a diagnosis, doctors sent Grace home with additional prescriptions of morphine. Her condition continued to worsen. Soon, she could no longer dress herself, sit, walk, or use the toilet on her own. Her parents had to move in to help with these tasks.

Grace, a doctor of chiropractic medicine, desperately longed to do research on her condition. The swelling of her brain, however, made it impossible for her eyes to track. She was unable to read and had no way to find answers. Her days were spent idle, lying on the couch, the pain subdued by morphine. She was limited to an existence of staring at the ceiling. At a loss for answers, doctors continued to renew her morphine prescription. After nine months from the onset of the illness with still no diagnosis or treatment in sight, Grace slipped into a world of darkness and depression.

Almost a year had gone by when, during a visit, a friend recognized her symptoms. Despite the apparent cure of her Lyme disease, Grace's symptoms resembled, her friend was certain, a less common manifestation of Lyme disease. Lyme radiculoneuritis is caused by *Borrelia burgdorferi* bacteria, with the infection finding safe harbor in the spinal cord and nerve roots. It is a neurological disease resulting in intense nerve pain, which radiates from the spine to the related limbs and organs.

Understanding that *Borrelia burgdorferi* bacteria were indeed still the underlying cause of her suffering, Grace finally had a direction to pursue. At this point, she refused to undergo another intravenous treatment of antibiotics. The antibiotics had been a deeply intrusive and unsuccessful attempt at killing off the Lyme bacteria in her body. Although she appeared to have improved some at the time of the treatment, it had left her depleted and ultimately still very sick. Instead, Grace clung to the hope of finding another way to regain her health. She learned of plant-based antibiotics and naturopathic treatments specific to Lyme disease. Filled with hope, Grace began taking these remedies. But at this point she had become so ill––more or less just hanging on to her existence––that it was hard to discern if the herbal remedies produced any results.

But one day this changed. Through a network of friends, someone had learned about her condition. This person had a relative who had recovered from bacterial Lyme meningitis through the use of a hyperbaric oxygen chamber.

Clinging to each straw, Grace decided to try the chamber. She was unable to drive, but her mother gave her a ride to her first experience with a hyperbaric oxygen chamber. The long trip was torturous for her aching body. But Grace remembers this first treatment well. Something definitely happened during that treatment. Something shifted and awoke in her body: nothing else had felt like it before. Finally––there was hope.

While longing for more treatments with the chamber, it was clear that driving the distance to where the hyperbaric chamber was located was too painful for Grace to endure. The ride was too long, the seating position in the car too agonizing. But nothing else she had tried had made a significant difference. Something had shifted in her body while in that chamber. It was her best shot. It had been a year since Grace had been able to work.

Without the ability to do any research, she spontaneously took out a bank loan and purchased a hyperbaric chamber. The chamber was placed in her home, and Grace immediately began daily treatments. Her parents had to assist her in getting in and out of the chamber. Seeing how difficult it was for Grace, her father built her a railing leading into the chamber.

And then something astounding took place. After only two weeks of daily hyperbaric treatments, her parents were able to go home. Grace had recovered enough that she could walk, dress, and go to the bathroom by herself. She could cook and eat again without help.

Gradually, she improved. Her ability to read, to focus, and to do research returned. She was able to learn and understand how the chamber functions and how it assisted in recovering her health. With these improvements her spirits rose and her depression left. As soon as she was able to drive safely, she started working again. At that point, she moved the chamber into her practice, so that her patients could benefit from it as well.

Dr. Grace Johnstone attributes the fact that she is here today and feeling better than ever to the benefits of hyperbaric oxygen treatments. She has regained her strength fully and is visibly bursting with energy and vitality. She has not forgotten, however, the arduous road of recovery and what finally turned the page from disease back to health.

While a patient is ill, commuting to receive treatments can be a real challenge and is often impossible, as Grace herself experienced. Yet, recognizing the importance of this treatment modality, she made it her mission to make affordable hyperbaric care available throughout the state of Vermont and created HyperbaricVermont.org, a nonprofit organization, which offers affordable hyperbaric oxygen therapy at various treatment sites. The organization focuses on training physicians and other healthcare providers to set up their own hyperbaric treatment chambers.

Thanks to HyperbaricVermont.org there are already several physicians in the state of Vermont who offer the treatment. The organization's informative website lists many research articles and has links to videos about the hyperbaric chamber and its treatment results. The website further includes an index that lists medical conditions that have been shown to benefit from hyperbaric treatments.

Dr. Grace Johnstone can be reached at hyperbaricvermont.org.

THE HYPERBARIC OXYGEN CHAMBER AND LYME DISEASE

The hyperbaric oxygen chamber is a pressurized tent-like space in which patients are treated with oxygen. Most often, monoplace––single use chambers––are being used. Multiplace chambers, which can treat multiple patients simultaneously, are more commonly used in hospital settings. The patient spends a given amount of time inside the chamber, breathing concentrated oxygen.

Treatments with the hyperbaric oxygen chamber counteract disease in a number of ways. During hyperbaric treatment, air pressure in the chamber is increased so that the patient breathes concentrated oxygen. Under higher atmospheric pressure, not only red blood cells but also the body's plasma is being loaded with oxygen. All fluids in the body are oxygenated, including spinal fluid, joint fluid, and fluid in the gut. Through these fluids, oxygen treatments work holistically. The fluids reach places in the body where the immune system can best build up its own defense. And with the increased, high level, anti-microbial oxygen in the plasma, it becomes difficult for the bacteria to hide.

One of its biggest attributes is its natural anti-microbial quality: pathogens favor low levels of oxygen. In laboratories, scientists intentionally create hypoxic environments to experiment with and learn from disease. Lyme bacteria also survive in low levels of oxygen. If exposed to high levels, the bacteria will die. This is the reason why the clever bacteria encapsulate, gather in protective biofilms, or burrow deeply into tissue where there is little or no blood supply––and therefore little oxygen. Typically, medication is transported through our oxygen-rich bloodstream, making these low-oxygen hiding places, including the brain, extremely hard to treat.

The body's oxygenated fluids are also highly anti-inflammatory. Since Lyme bacteria themselves cause inflammation wherever they choose to reside and trigger immune system inflammatory responses, the anti-inflammatory quality of the oxygenated fluids is crucial to addressing Lyme disease.

Furthermore, hyperbaric treatments normalize the immune function: Lyme spirochetes are incredibly intelligent and have various weapons with which to fight natural, healthy immune responses. On one side, the bacteria aggravate the immune system and so make it hyperactive. This hyperactivity can cause the immune system to attack itself in an effort to eliminate the intruder, while not recognizing that it is engaging in a self-destructive response. On the other side, the bacteria suppress immune response: the immune system therefore cannot detect the intruder, and so the bacteria can go about their business undiscovered. Oxygen treatments help the immune system get back to normal functioning, allowing it to realize the presence of microbes and successfully eliminate these intruders while abstaining from self-destructive actions.

Oxygen treatments are not entirely new. Before we had modern medical equipment, physicians sent their wealthy patients to the sea to recover from chronic and stubborn illnesses. It was known that sea air was conducive to regaining one's health. By the edge of the sea, at a level of zero altitude, patients would stay and rest for several weeks or months while breathing sea air. Many eventually recuperated from their illness. Without knowing the scientific reasons behind the cure, these physicians were already working with a treatment method that underlies the concept of the hyperbaric oxygen chamber. Air at sea level causes oxygen to easily pass through lung membranes into the blood. The atmospheric pressure is much higher at sea level—about 14.7 pounds per square inch. At high altitude, where the air pressure is much lower, it is more difficult for oxygen to enter the vascular system. The hyperbaric chamber imitates and intensifies an environment high in atmospheric pressure.

While in the United States hyperbaric chamber treatments still fall into the experimental treatment category for most illnesses including treatments for Lyme disease, other countries have embraced this treatment modality decades ago. Their health care providers have administered millions of hyperbaric treatment sessions over this timespan. The number of available research articles ranks in the thousands.

Examples of Hyperbaric Treatments

Oxygen treatments stimulate the brain and nervous system to heal in previously unknown ways. After an insult to the brain (meningitis, anoxia, brain injury or trauma, stroke, etc.) where there is resulting cell death, the surrounding neurons are often alive but not working properly. They are in a state of limbo and are referred to as "idling neurons" –– not dead, but not functioning. Oxygen therapy changes the metabolism in these cells to jumpstart them so they can come back online. Studies with hyperbaric oxygen treatments show that in some cases this can happen even years after the event!

For Lyme disease, revitalizing neurons is crucial beyond the mere elimination of bacteria. An immune system and physiology rattled by the intrusion of a long-term bacterial attack will need to regain its resilience after the bacteria have been eliminated. Hyperbaric oxygen treatments help to regain neuroplasticity and healthy brain and tissue function.

It is commonly accepted that we will suffer from aching joints or forgetfulness after we reach a certain age. Aging is mostly a chronic low-grade inflammatory process––a degenerative inflammatory condition––affecting one area or another in the body. With hyperbaric oxygen treatments, we have a tool to fight inflammation holistically, throughout the body, while addressing acute and chronic conditions without side effects.

Inflammation in the body is also caused by vigorous athletic pursuits or simple overuse of the body. Athletes know this well. Many top-ranked athletes use hyperbaric oxygen treatments for recovery––some even have a chamber at home.

Herxing and Hyperbaric Treatments

A successful hyperbaric treatment for bacteria-caused illnesses will result in the dying off of bacteria. This can, in some cases, be traumatic for the system and result in a Jarisch-Herxheimer reaction (often simply referred to as a Herxheimer reaction or herxing) which needs to be monitored closely. Because herxing is a serious side effect, I have dedicated a separate chapter to this topic.

Due to the possibility of herxing, hyperbaric treatments need to be started slowly and monitored closely, and the detox process supported, if necessary, with homeopathic medicines or plant-based herbs and tinctures.

In addition to successfully treating Lyme disease patients with hyperbaric treatments, Dr. Johnstone discovered that herxing from hyperbaric treatments can also serve as an important diagnostic tool. After she moved the hyperbaric chamber to her office, Dr. Johnstone began treating patients with oxygen for various chronic, non-bacterial conditions, such as MS, Parkinson's, ALS, vertigo, rheumatoid arthritis, trigeminal neuralgia, and traumatic brain injuries. Hyperbaric treatments have been shown to be helpful for these conditions. What was really surprising and fascinating to Dr. Johnstone, however, was that many of these patients suffering from these chronic illnesses experienced a Herxheimer reaction during hyperbaric treatment. The reason for a Herxheimer reaction is a die-off from systemic infection––dying bacteria. With these chronic conditions, a die-off of bacteria would *not* be expected to occur, as the illnesses are not considered to be caused by bacteria. With hyperbaric treatments, combined with proper detox support, many of Dr. Johnstone's patients gradually recuperated and, eventually, no longer suffered from their chronic disease. This was a clear indication that the original cause of the illness was actually bacterial––Lyme disease and other bacterial infections—mirroring non-bacterial diseases.

✳

You can see how hyperbaric oxygen treatments can assist in pinpointing the origin of a disease. Lyme disease can be incredibly difficult to diagnose, as tissue damaged by bacteria causes symptoms similar to other neurological, nonbacterial diseases.

Multiples Sclerosis (MS) is a good example. When Lyme bacteria consume the myelin sheaths of neurons in the brain, an MRI (magnetic resonance imaging) will show demyelination. Demyelination is also one of the symptoms and a major diagnostic indicator for MS. From the MRI image, it is not possible to detect if the demyelination is a sign of MS or the result of raging Lyme bacteria. But if an MS patient responds positively—showing a Herxheimer reaction or improving—to hyperbaric oxygen treatment, it is an indication that demyelination diagnosed as MS may have indeed been caused by bacteria.

Recent studies with the use of MRI show *re*myelination after exposure to hyperbaric treatments. This is very exciting and something that we did not know was even possible!

✳

Whether Dr. Johnstone's patients with chronic illnesses (other than Lyme disease) experienced a Herxheimer response from hyperbaric oxygen treatments or started to improve after treatments even though they didn't herx, she noted a positive response to treatment. Intrigued, Dr. Johnstone tested these patients for possible Lyme disease. *All* of these patients tested positive! Treatment was then adjusted to target Lyme disease specifically, and these patients gradually improved. Eventually, many no longer suffered from the chronic condition they thought they had. Some of them had been ill for decades, yet were able to recover completely.

Other Treatments

"Within each of us
lies the power of our consent to health and sickness,
to riches and poverty, to freedom and to slavery.
It is we who control these, and not another."

--Richard Bach

There are of course many other treatment methods used in healing Lyme disease than those described here. With the steady increase and epidemic character of this disease, it is to be expected that there will be additional knowledge gained about the bacteria and how it operates in the body, which inevitably will lead to treatment methods yet to be developed.

Several other protocols in addition to those mentioned in this book, including homeopathic remedies, additional tinctures and supplements, Chinese herbs, vitamin C infusions, just to mention a few, have been used by practitioners and may be worth investigating.

In a recent study at the Department of Molecular Microbiology and Immunology, Johns Hopkins University, out of thirty-five essential oils tested, ten showed significant killing activity against *Borrelia burgdorferi* bacteria. Five of these oils, specifically oils from garlic bulbs, allspice berries, myrrh trees, spiked ginger lily blossoms, and may chang fruit, successfully killed all laboratory cultures of Lyme bacteria. Twenty-one days after the Lyme bacteria were killed off, no further bacteria regrew.

These experiments are very promising, but they are the result of tests done in laboratories. Lyme spirochetes are extremely intelligent and adaptable. What works in a petri dish does not necessarily work in a human body. We will be on the lookout for future developments.

How long should a patient stay on a protocol?

For long-term chronic Lyme disease, one and a half years to three years of constant pressure might be necessary to eliminate the bacteria's presence in the body. For Lyme disease in its early stages, six months to a year and a half may suffice. Bacteria are smart and constantly engaged in adapting to their environment. Alternating treatment methods is one way to keep them at bay. After Lyme symptoms have disappeared, it does not hurt to follow up periodically with a short protocol.

Nutrition and Diet

"When diet is wrong, medicine is of no use.
When diet is correct, medicine is of no need."

--Ayurvedic Proverb

Nutrition can greatly assist in the healing process and help restore damage done by bacteria. A healthy diet supports the immune system and has tremendous effect on body, mind, and spirit. Here are a few Lyme-specific suggestions:

Lyme spirochetes prefer the collagen of their host, which is present throughout the body. In order to digest it, the bacteria release a substance--their poop--which breaks down these molecules. Once broken down, the collagen become nutrients for the spirochetes. Bone broth and gelatin are collagen-rich foods and help restore these tissues in our bodies.

Bacteria feed on sugar. We want to starve them. Therefore, it is a good idea to minimize the intake of sugar, especially any refined sugars. Abstain from eating refined flour and grains for a while to make it harder for bacteria to feed. Supplement fruits with nuts and seeds. You don't need to be a purist, however. A little raw honey or maple syrup is always good for the soul.

During and after a round of antibiotics, the intestinal flora becomes compromised. Probiotics can help restore the gut biome and hence decrease inflammation. Fermented foods such as sauerkraut and kimchi contain high amounts of enzymes and aid in the restoration and maintenance of the intestinal flora.

Oregano oil has many health benefits. Among others, it is said to be anti-inflammatory, anti-viral, and anti-parasitic. Some folks have had good results with oregano oil taken internally or put directly on the tick bite.

If choosing between coffee and tea, choose tea. Coffee can be hard on the adrenal glands, which are the root of all bodily functions. We want the adrenals to be strong and healthy in order to deal with the challenges in our bodily environment. Coffee can drain the adrenals and hence cause even greater fatigue, the opposite of what most of us seek in coffee.

Best to stay away from alcohol consumption, recreational drugs, and activities that cause stress. The body needs all its energy to heal when sick.

NATIVE AMERICAN METHODS

"Walking is man's best medicine."

--Hippocrates

When Europeans returned from their explorations to the New World, they brought with them not only knowledge of new places and scores of traded and stolen goods, but also a terrible disease--syphilis. Europe was entirely unprepared for this horrific illness. They had never seen anything like it up until the time when Columbus returned from the New World. While it is difficult to prove the exact origin of syphilis, and some scholars argue that syphilis may have existed previously in Europe but had gone unrecognized, only exhumed skeletons from the time after Columbus show syphilitic damage.

Europeans were at a loss as to how to treat this new and devastating illness, which quickly began to spread like wildfire. They called it the "French disease" because the first recorded outbreak occurred in 1494/1495 in Naples, Italy, during a French invasion. Monks who usually knew what to do were just as much at a loss as were the old crones, who had the handed down knowledge of every herb and its healing property within range. Neither did the blessed healing oils from the Church, nor the protective saints seem to have any effect on the disease. Syphilis raged in Europe.

Not until wealthy syphilitics returned to the Caribbean Islands, did they find some relief. Natives of the islands understood how to treat infections caused by syphilis spirochetes. They used a combination of lifestyle changes and remedies that included sweat baths, strenuous exercise, a special diet, and herbs.

The use of sweat lodges and steam baths was not invented by the natives of the Caribbean Islands. The tradition goes back to the Stone Age. Hunters and gatherers already understood the benefit of heat. Through observation they knew that a fever could cure a disease. In an attempt to simulate a fever, they induced sweating either by external heat, through sweat lodges and steam baths, or through heat- and sweat-producing herbal teas. Put in simple terms, they observed that sweating flushes sickness out of the body.

Sweat lodges were a common remedy on the Caribbean Islands as part of the cure for syphilis infections. In combination with sweat baths, natives prescribed a concoction made from the resin of the guaiacum tree, a tree that inhabits the entire Caribbean region. They also demanded hard physical exercise from their patients in order to activate the lymphatic system and blood circulation. And finally, they required their patients to hold off from heavy food and to stick to a very light diet during recovery.

Syphilis and Lyme disease are both relapsing infections caused by spirochetes. Syphilis bacteria are in fact close cousins to Lyme spirochetes. Often, Lyme disease is referred to as "deer syphilis," as the diseases are so similar in many ways. Wolf D. Storl, the author of *Healing Lyme Disease Naturally*, speculated that the protocol natives of the Caribbean Islands used to cure syphilis could very well cure Lyme disease.

Borrelia burgdorferi bacteria, like the syphilis bacteria, thrive at a temperature of 96.8°F--our ideal body temperature. Today we understand that fever is a natural defense reaction of the body against infection. We know also that at a temperature of 107.6°F (42°C) spirochetes are being killed off effectively.

Luckily, we have the ability to take saunas where sweat lodges or steam baths are unavailable. (Warning: heat therapy is not advisable for everyone. Although the artificially created heat of saunas, sweat lodges, or steam baths is external heat and does not reflect the body temperature, an internal body temperature of 107.6°F (42°C) would be extremely dangerous! Check with your health practitioner prior to using heat therapy.)

The natural remedy guaiacum, which the natives used, is hard to find these days. Teasel, a kidney and liver cleanser, can be used as a supportive tincture instead. It is readily available and has proven to be an effective replacement for guaiacum in the process of healing Lyme.

The natives of the islands prescribed a diet of only white foods, such as white beans and white potatoes for their syphilis patients. A light diet frees energy from the digestive process, making energy available to the healing process. Recent studies have shown that lots of protein, fast foods, and refined sugars raise the acidity of blood and tissue. Hyperacidity is an ideal environment for disease. To keep acidity low, a bland diet of mainly fresh and natural foods––lots of fresh fruit and vegetables––is recommended, spiked with occasional sour foods––pickles, sauerkraut, sourdough bread, etc. Alcohol, salt, and spices should be avoided during recovery.

In between rests, the healers of the Caribbean Islands ordered their patients to do hard physical labor. When not resting in their hammocks, the wealthy but sick Europeans, not used to physical labor, were ordered to chop wood to regain their health. History tells of several thousand Spanish syphilitics that were cured of syphilis by the strict protocol of the natives of the Caribbean Islands.

When afflicted with Lyme disease, finding the right balance between hard physical exercise and the necessary rest is similar to walking a razor's edge. Hard physical exercise induces healthy sweating, encourages blood circulation, and stimulates the immune defense system. Yet too much can cause relapsing and setbacks.

A Quick Word on Vaccines

Attempts at Lyme disease vaccines in the past unfortunately had questionable results. Although the assertion was never subject to any testing, it was alleged that the SmithKline Beecham vaccine on the market in the 1990s caused more Lyme disease than it prevented. Some people who had received the vaccine began to develop arthritis. A lawsuit was filed and the vaccine was removed from the market.

In 2017 the Food and Drug Administration approved a Fast Track designation for a new Lyme disease vaccine. Initial trials were completed in 2018 and the vaccine is currently in phase II trials. It could possibly be on the market within five years.

HERXHEIMER REACTION

"What remains in diseases after the
crisis is apt to produce relapses."

––Hippocrates

The reason why we choose to take antibiotics or herbs, or employ other treatment methods is to kill off the bacteria that have invaded our body and caused inflammation. If the chosen treatment is successful, there will be a large die-off of these bacterial organisms. Decomposing bacteria, and the substances they create while decomposing, are toxic to our system.

Toxic bacterial fragments float around in the body before they are flushed out. In about fifteen percent of all patients these dead organisms and toxins can be overwhelming to the bodily system. This can, in some cases, cause a severe reaction called a Jarisch-Herxheimer reaction (often simply referred to as a Herxheimer reaction or herxing) which needs to be monitored closely. The toxins can be particularly hard on the liver, gallbladder, or lymphatic system.

A Herxheimer reaction can be confusing for the patient who experiences it, as patients may conclude that the disease is getting worse. Experiencing more and worse symptoms shortly after the beginning of a treatment can easily give the impression that the wrong treatment is being used. In reality, these patients are actually on the right track. Practitioners often look for a Herxheimer reaction. It is essentially a good indicator that treatment is working and that a patient is heading in the right direction.

Usually, a Herxheimer reaction occurs within the first month or two of treatment. Sometimes a Herxheimer reaction will set in later on, when prescriptions or herbs are changed, or a new antibiotic is tried.

When a Herxheimer reaction occurs, it is important to assist the body with the flushing out of the dead spirochete fragments. A good detoxing protocol quickly aids in lessening unwanted, sometimes severe symptoms. Some Herxheimer reactions are, however, barely noticeable.

Not experiencing a Herxheimer reaction does not indicate that treatment is not working. As previously mentioned, only a few patients actually do experience this very uncomfortable reaction. It is not something that has to occur to confirm that a given treatment is successful.

Final Thoughts on Treatments for Lyme Disease

"Health is the greatest gift."

—Buddha

It cannot be overemphasized that each patient has a unique immune-system and a unique history of illnesses and injuries. Therefore, each person responds differently to bacterial infections. There is no one treatment that fits all, no one pharmaceutical drug or herb that can cure all Lyme disease patients. For each afflicted person, the treatment protocol may vary and may even need to be adjusted multiple times.

Each person may feel differently about using a certain form of treatment. If antibiotics are preferred, then they should be chosen. If a nonconventional treatment is preferred, that avenue should be taken. At other times, a combination of antibiotics and herbs may be the ideal choice of treatment.

It is tremendously helpful to collaborate with a skilled practitioner who is trained and experienced in treating Lyme disease. To have a practitioner accompany you along the uncertain road of recuperation can be beneficial in so many ways. Besides monitoring treatment and progress, the practitioner also serves as a valuable observer. Once infected with Lyme disease, it can be very hard to detect any progress. The mind becomes foggy and emotions run low. Depression darkens any positive outlook on the future. Energy and stamina are phenomena of the past. A practitioner can lend support based on objective observation of the recuperation process and can give encouragement and hope when the road seems rough and the disease appears never to improve.

And finally, developments in herbal as well as antibiotic treatments for Lyme disease are not static. Treatments change all the time. New pharmaceuticals are constantly developed and new plants discovered that can aid in the healing process of Lyme disease. In essence, treating Lyme disease is still an experimental process.

GRATITUDE

"Being grateful is not only the greatest of virtues,
but is also the parent of all other virtues."

--Cicero (106-43 BCE)

One would think that nothing good can come from being infected with Lyme disease. The disease changes our body, our mind, and our psyche. But maybe there are, hidden within these changes, a chance of hope and a glimmer of light.

Just as the spirochetes that enter our body are not the same ones that leave our body, we are not the same once we reemerge from this disease. It will have changed us in a number of ways. It most certainly will have given us the compassion for others who suffer from Lyme disease. It will have forced us to slow down. And with slowing down, we may have noticed a world much different from the one we are used to. And, ultimately, the disease turns our outlook inward, where we may discover aspects of ourselves we have so far been unaware of.

When we reemerge from Lyme with a clear mind and a spirit high, rediscovering the beauty and preciousness of each day, we truly have been given a gift.

I wish with all my heart that if you are inflicted by Lyme disease, or if you know someone who is, that my story and the chapters in this book will be of help. My hope is that you may experience the same positive and terrific results that I have. Should the disease have debilitated you, I wish that you may find again the vitality and joy you once had.

BIBLIOGRAPHY

Buhner, Stephen Harrod. Stephen Buhner answers Questions about his Herbal Protocols for Lyme Disease and Co-Infections. http://buhnerhealinglyme.com/ (visited January 2019)

Buhner, Stephen Harrod. *Healing Lyme*. Silver City, NM: Raven Press, 2015.

Butler, Thomas. "The Jarisch–Herxheimer Reaction After Antibiotic Treatment of Spirochetal Infections: A Review of Recent Cases and Our Understanding of Pathogenesis" *The American Society of Tropical Medicine and Hygiene.* 2017. https://www.ncbi.nlm.nih.gov/pmc/articles/PMC5239707/ (last visited October 2019)

Chien-YuHuang, Yen-WenChen, Tseng-HuiKao, Hsin-KuoKao, Yu-ChinLee, Jui-ChunCheng, Jia-HorngWang. "Hyperbaric oxygen therapy as an effective adjunctive treatment for chronic Lyme disease," May 2014. https://www.sciencedirect.com/science/article/pii/S1726490114000422 (visited October 2018)

"Cleve Backster's Pflanzenexperimente," last modified in 2013, http://www.quantec.eu (visited June 2016)

Cline JC. "Nutritional aspects of detoxification in clinical practice." Altern Ther Health Med. 2015 May-Jun;21(3):54-62.

https://www.ncbi.nlm.nih.gov/pubmed/26026145 (last visited October 2019)

DiBiase, Florence. "Education on Tick Bites, Tick Borne Disease, and Prevention in Middlebury, VT." 2017. http://scholarworks.uvm.edu/fmclerk (visited June 2018)

"Essential Oils from Garlic and other Herbs and Spices kill "Persister" Lyme Disease Bacteria." Johns Hopkins University Bloomberg School of Public Health. December 3, 2018. https://www.sciencedaily.com/releases/2018/12/181203115443.htm (visited January 2019)

Farhi, D; Dupin, N (Sep–Oct 2010). "Origins of syphilis and management in the immunocompetent patient: facts and controversies". *Clinics in Dermatology.* 28 (5): 533–38. doi:10.1016/j.clindermatol.2010.03.011. PMID 20797514. https://www.ncbi.nlm.nih.gov/pubmed/20797514 (last visited October 2019)

Feng Jie. Shi Wanliang. Miklossy Judith. Tauxe Genevieve M.. McMeniman Conor J.. Zhang Ying. "Identification of Essential Oils with Strong Activity against Stationary Phase Borrelia burgdorferi" *Antibiotics* 2018, 7(4), 89; https://doi.org/10.3390/antibiotics7040089 (visited April 2019)

Hermann, Ecki. "Wir sind ein Hochrisikogebiet." April 3, 2018. Liechtensteiner Vaterland.

Hermann, Ecki. "Zecken – kleine Tierchen, grosse Wirkung." April 4, 2018. Liechtensteinische Ärztekammer, Schaan.

"History of Lyme Disease," https://www.bayarealyme.org/about-lyme/history-lyme/disease/ (last visited March 15, 2019)

"How many people get Lyme disease?" Center for Disease Control and Prevention, (last reviewed December 21, 2018) https://www.cdc.gov/lyme/stats/humancases.html (last visited October 30, 2019)

Hirokazu Ueda, Yukio Kikuta, and Kazuhiko Matsuda, "Plant communication"

Plant Signal Behav. 2012 Feb 1; 7(2): 222–226. https://www.ncbi.nlm.nih.gov/pmc/articles/PMC3405699/ (last visited October 30, 2019)

Hokynar, Kati. "*Chlamydia*-Like Organisms (CLOs) in Finnish *Ixodes ricinus* Ticks and Human Skin" *Microorganisms*. 2016 Sep; 4(3): 28. Published online 2016 Aug 18. doi: 10.3390/microorganisms4030028 https://www.ncbi.nlm.nih.gov/pmc/articles/PMC5039588/ (last visited October 2019)

Holland, Kimberly. "How Close Are We to Getting a Lyme Disease Vaccine?" Healthline Media. June 6, 2019 https://www.healthline.com/health-news/lyme-disease-vaccine-update#A-new-option-to-stop-Lyme-disease (last visited October 2019)

"Hyperbaric oxygen therapy" Mayo Foundation for Medical Education and Research (MFMER)

https://www.mayoclinic.org/tests-procedures/hyperbaric-oxygen-therapy/about/pac-20394380 (last visited October 2019)

Hyperbaric Vermont–Oxygen Therapy. "Research & Resources" (last modified 2019) https://www.hyperbaricvermont.org/research-resources/ (visited May 2019)

Hyperbaric Vermont – Oxygen Therapy. "Hyperbaric Vermont; changing lives through hyperbaric oxygen therapy."

(last updated 2019) https://www.hyperbaricvermont.org/ (visited July 2019)

Jie Feng, Wanliang Shi, Judith Miklossy, Genevieve M. Tauxe, Conor J. McMeniman and Ying Zhang. "Identification of Essential Oils with Strong Activity against Stationary Phase Borrelia burgdorferi." October 16, 2018. *Antibiotics* 2018, 7(4), 89; https://doi.org/10.3390/antibiotics7040089 (visited April 2019)

Jonas, Julian. "Dementia and Alzheimer's Disease." December 17, 2017. http://www.centerforhomeopathy.com/blog/2017/12/17/dementia-and-alzheimers-disease (visited August 2018)

Jonas, Julian. "A Case of Lyme Disease." September, 22, 2017. http://www.centerforhomeopathy.com/blog/2017/9/22/a-case-of-lyme-disease (visited August 2018)

Jonas, Julian. "Treating Lyme Disease with Homeopathy." September 22, 2017. http://www.centerforhomeopathy.com/blog/2017/9/22/treating-lyme-disease-with-homeopathy (visited August 2018)

Klass, Perri, M.D. "The Challenge of Diagnosing Lyme Disease" (July 29, 2019) https://www.nytimes.com/2019/07/29/well/family/the-challenge-of-diagnosing-lyme-disease.html (visited July 29, 2019)

Klein AV, Kiat H. "Detox diets for toxin elimination and weight management: a critical review of the evidence." National Center for Biotechnology Information, U.S. National Library of Medicine, J Hum Nutr Diet. 2015 Dec;28(6):675-86. doi: 10.1111/jhn.12286. Epub 2014 Dec 18. https://www.ncbi.nlm.nih.gov/pubmed/25522674 (last visited October 2019)

Li T, Ito A, Chen X, Long C, Okamoto M, Raoul F, Giraudoux P, Yanagida T, Nakao M, Sako Y, Xiao N, Craig PS. "Usefulness of pumpkin seeds combined with areca nut extract in community-based treatment of human taeniasis in northwest Sichuan Province, China." Acta Trop. 2012 Nov;124(2):152-7. doi: 10.1016/j.actatropica.2012.08.002. Epub 2012 Aug 11. National Center for Biotechnology Information, U.S. National Library of Medicine https://www.ncbi.nlm.nih.gov/pubmed/22910218 (last visited October 2019)

Lindl, Jim. *Mr. Teasel My Hero*. Montana, USA: The Teasel Foundation, 2016.

LymeMD. "Biofilms: hyperbaric?" July 22, 2013, http://lymemd.blogspot.com/2013/07/biofilms-hyperbaric.html (visited October 12, 2018)

MacDonald, Alan B. to Speak in DC on Lyme and Nematodes, (May 19, 2016) "Lyme Bacteria Hides Inside Parasitic Worms, Causing Chronic Brain Diseases" http://www.mvlymecenter.org/2016/05/19/alan-b-macdonald-to-speak-in-dc-on-lyme-and-nematodes/ (visited May 2019)

Masatsugu Toyota, Dirk Spencer, Satoe Sawai-Toyota, Wang Jiaqi, Tong Zhang, Abraham J. Koo, Gregg A. Howe, Simon Gilroy, "Glutamate triggers long-distance, calcium-based plant defense signaling" *Science* 14 Sep 2018:Vol. 361, Issue 6407, pp. 1112-1115

Mayo Foundation for Medical Education and Research (MFMER). "Lyme Disease." https://www.mayoclinic.org/diseases-conditions/lyme-disease/symptoms-causes/syc-20374651 (last visited October 2019)

Mudd Austin T., Berding Kirsten, Wang Mei, Donovan Sharon M., Dilger Ryan N., University of Illinois College of Agricultural, Consumer and Environmental Sciences. "Serum cortisol mediates the relationship between fecal Ruminococcus and brain N-acetylaspartate in the young pig." *Gut Microbes*, 2017; 1 DOI: 10.1080/19490976.2017.1353849, (August 21, 2017) https://www.sciencedaily.com/releases/2017/08/170821122736.htm (visited May 2019)

Newby, Kris. "The secret Swiss Agent: Puzzling comments reveal new twist to the Lyme disease saga." October 13, 2016. https://scopeblog.stanford.edu/2016/10/13/the-secret-swiss-agent-puzzling-comments-reveal-new-twist-to-lyme-disease-sage/ (visited January 10, 2019)

Nordqvist, Joseph. (December 18, 2017) "Health benefits of Gingko biloba"

https://www.medicalnewstoday.com/articles/263105.php (last visited November 2019)

O'Neil, Dennis. "Adapting to High Altitude" Human Biological Adaptability. https://www2.palomar.edu/anthro/adapt/adapt_3.htm (last visited October 2019)

"Oxygen Levels at Altitude" Center for Wilderness Safety Inc. https://www.wildsafe.org/resources/outdoor-safety-101/altitude-safety-101/high-altitude-oxygen-levels/ (last visited October 2019)

Peere, Wendy. "Protein Study Shows Evolutionary Link between Plants, Humans," last modified February 15, 2010, http://purdue.edu (visited November 2018)

Pennisi Elizabeth, *Science,* Sep. 13, 2018 "Plants communicate distress using their own kind of nervous system" https://www.sciencemag.org/news/2018/09/plants-communicate-distress-using-their-own-kind-nervous-system (last visited October 2019)

Piller, Charles. "The 'Swiss Agent': Long-forgotten research unearths new mystery about Lyme disease." October 12, 2016. https://www.statnews.com/2016/10/12/swiss-agent-lyme-disease-mystery/ (visited July 3, 2018)

Pompa, Daniel. "141: Could Parasites Be Making You Sick?" (November 4, 2016) https://drpompa.com/podcasts/141-could-parasites-be-making-you-sick/ (visited May 2019)

"Pumpkin Seeds for Parasites and Intestinal Worms" Superfood Profiles. (2018) https://superfoodprofiles.com/pumpkin-seeds-parasites-intestinal-worms (visited May 2019)

Rocky Mountain Laboratories Microscopy Branch, National Institute of Allergy and Infectious Diseases, National Institutes of Health, Hamilton, Montana 59840, USA. "The antimicrobial agent melittin exhibits powerful in vitro inhibitory effects on the Lyme disease spirochete." July 25, 1997. https://www.ncbi.nlm.nih.gov/pubmed/9233664 (visited January 2019)

Rose, Amber. "Innovative effects of bee venom therapy on Lyme disease: A pioneering study." 4th International Conference and Exhibition on Immunology, September 28-30, 2015 Houston, Texas, USA, https://immunology.conferenceseries.com/abstract/2015/innovative-effects-of-bee-venom-therapy-on-lyme-disease-a-pioneering-study (visited January 2019)

Scott, Timothy Lee. *Invasive Plant Medicine*. Rochester, VT: Healing Arts Press, 2010.

Severson, Stephanie. "Parasites - Often Hidden and Undiagnosed." (March 29, 2011) https://ezinearticles.com/?Parasites---Often-Hidden-and-Undiagnosed&id=6127689 (visited May 2019)

Storl, Wolf D. *Healing Lyme Disease Naturally*. Berkeley, CA: North Atlantic Books, 2007.

"The History of the Lyme Disease Vaccine." The History of Vaccines – An Educational Resource by the College of Physicians of Philadelphia https://www.historyofvaccines. org/content/articles/history-lyme-disease-vaccine (last visited October 2019)

Tompkins, Peter, and Bird, Christopher. *Das Geheime Leben der Pflanzen*. Frankfurt am Main, Deutschland: Fischer Taschenbuch GmbH, 1997.

"Transmission of Parasitic Diseases." Center for Disease Control and Prevention. (February 21, 2018) https://www. cdc.gov/parasites/transmission/index.html (visited May 2019)

VPR Podcast on Tick Population in Vermont, 2018. http:// digital.vpr.net/post/addison-county-tick-population-doubles-last-year#stream/0 (visited January 2019)

Walter, Katharine. "Climate change is speeding up the spread of Lyme disease," July 1, 2016. https://statnews. com/2016/07/01/lyme-disease-climate-change/ (visited May 2017)

"What Causes MS?" The National Multiple Sclerosis Society https://www.nationalmssociety.org/What-is-MS/What-Causes-MS (last visited October 2019)

"What you need to know about *Borrelia mayonii*" Centers for Disease Control and Prevention, National Center for Emerging and Zoonotic Infectious Diseases (NCEZID), Division of Vector-Borne Diseases (DVBD) https://www.cdc.gov/lyme/mayonii/index.html?CDC_AA_refVal=https%3A%2F%2Fwww.cdc.gov%2Fticks%2Fmayonii.html (last visited October 2019)

ABOUT THE AUTHOR

Isabella (Isa) S. Oehry was born and raised in the Principality of Liechtenstein, a small country sandwiched between Austria and Switzerland. After finishing her education in Europe and then traveling and ski racing throughout the United States, Isa eventually settled in Vermont. She continued her education, earning a degree in management information systems. But her strong interest in the mystery of the human mind and our untapped potential prompted Isa to pursue an advanced degree in psychology, with a specialization in clinical mental health.

After contracting Lyme disease and undergoing unsuccessful treatment with antibiotics, Isa began extensive research seeking alternative healing modalities. Eventually she found what she was looking for and was able to fully recover. Realizing, however, how many people are afflicted by this debilitating disease while unaware of alternative options, Isa felt a strong desire to document her personal journey on how to heal Lyme disease beyond the use of antibiotics.

Isa is also the author of *Under A Blue Moon*, an insightful and humorous chronicle that challenges the reader to step outside the personal comfort zone and discover the secret powers of the mind. Today, she still lives in Vermont where she writes, works as an artist, keeps bees, organizes workshops, and hosts guests at her farm. She also considers herself fortunate to be the steward of an old cedar forest that contains blankets of magical mosses and countless fungi. You can see a trail map, pictures and documentation on the mosses and fungi on her website: www.isaoehry.com

APPENDIX

The remedies and supplements mentioned below are those that I have personally taken with great success. You should be able to purchase or order these through your local herbal and tincture supplier or your food co-op. The suggested dosages are the recommendations I followed and are listed for informational purposes only. These recommendations are not meant to serve as medical advice.

BASE TINCTURES:

Japanese Knotweed	(Polygonum cuspidatum)
Red Sage	(Salvia miltiorrhiza)
Chinese Scullcap	(Scutellaria baicalensis)

One teaspoon of each, in the form of a tincture, three times a day. (Can be mixed together into one convenient formula.) I continued with the base tinctures for a full two years.

After having taken the base tinctures for three months, I added one teaspoon of

Green Chiretta   (Andrographis)

in the form of a tincture, three times a day. (Warning: high likelihood of a Herxheimer reaction. Please read the information on Herxheimer reactions in Part III, Treatments. A Herxheimer reaction can be very unpleasant and potentially dangerous.)

IMMUNE SYSTEM BOOSTERS:

In order to assist my weakened immune system, I took the following supplements:

Selenium	(200 mcg/day)
Cat's claw	(1/2 tsp., 3 times a day)
Siberian ginseng	(1/2 tsp., 3 times a day)
Astragalus	(1 tsp., 3 times a day)
Vitamin C	(2000 mg/day)
Vitamin B complex	(daily as recommended)
Vitamin E	(800 IU/day)
Echinacea angustifolia	(1 tsp., 3 times a day)
Royal jelly	(1 tsp./day)
Zinc	(50 mg/day)
Copper	(3 mg/day)

After six months, I felt significantly stronger and let these supplements run out.

OTHER HEALING MODALITIES:

I also engaged in other healing modalities, including hyperbaric oxygen treatments, regular saunas, diet, and controlled exercise, which you can read about in Part III, Treatments.

Since our immune systems are unique, and each carries its own history, there is no guarantee that what worked for me will be the right remedy or combination for you. It is always best to embark on a healing journey under the guidance of a skilled practitioner.

Printed in the United States
By Bookmasters